Quarterly Essay

Quarterly Essay is published four times a year by Black Inc., an imprint of Schwartz Books Pty Ltd.
Publisher: Morry Schwartz.

ISBN 9781760643270 ISSN 1832-0953

Subscriptions – 1 year print & digital (4 issues): $79.95 within Australia incl. GST. Outside Australia $119.95. 2 years print & digital (8 issues): $149.95 within Australia incl. GST. 1 year digital only: $49.95.

Payment may be made by Mastercard or Visa, or by cheque made out to Schwartz Books. Payment includes postage and handling.

To subscribe, fill out and post the subscription card or form inside this issue, or subscribe online:

quarterlyessay.com
subscribe@blackincbooks.com
Phone: 61 3 9486 0288

Correspondence should be addressed to:

The Editor, Quarterly Essay
22–24 Northumberland Street
Collingwodd VIC 3066 Australia
Phone: 61 3 9486 0288 / Fax: 61 3 9011 6106
Email: quarterlyessay@blackincbooks.com

Editor: Chris Feik. Management: Elisabeth Young. Publicity: Anna Lensky. Design: Guy Mirabella. Assistant Editor: Kirstie Innes-Will. Production Coordinator: Marilyn de Castro. Typesetting: Tristan Main.

Printed in Australia by McPherson's Printing Group. The paper used to produce this book comes from wood grown in sustainable forests.

"We saw aspects of a mental health system that we had thought confined to history. Sadly, this was not the case."

—The Oakden Report: The report of the Oakden Review, SA Health, 2017

"Unsurprisingly, many of the reforms recommended in this Inquiry report have been proposed before."

—Productivity Commission, Inquiry Report into Mental Health, Vol. 1, 2020

"If history is any indication, reform will not be easy. Despite best endeavours, previous efforts to redesign the mental health system in Victoria, and across Australia more broadly, have not been realised. As a result, the state's mental health system has catastrophically failed to live up to expectations and is unprepared for current and future challenges. This persistent gap between the rhetoric of past inquiries and the reality for people living with mental illness or psychological distress ... has been described by some as devastating."

—Royal Commission into Victoria's Mental Health System, Final Report, Vol. 5, 2021

"The patient brings out of the armoury of the past the weapons with which he defends himself against the progress of the treatment – weapons which we must wrest from him one by one. We have learned that the patient repeats instead of remembering, and repeats under the conditions of resistance. We may now ask what it is that he in fact repeats or acts out ... we have to do our therapeutic work on it, which consists in a large measure in tracing it back to the past."

—Sigmund Freud, "Remembering, Repeating and Working-Through", 1914

"A strange picture and strange prisoners."
"No more strange than us," I said.

—Plato, The Republic

NOT WAVING, DROWNING

Mental illness and vulnerability in Australia

Sarah Krasnostein

"Australians today are a complacent people but our boast of living in a lucky country [is] at times just strident enough to betray that we cannot yet take our material comforts utterly for granted," wrote J.P. Parkinson, a psychiatrist, forty years ago in the *Australian and New Zealand Journal of Psychiatry*. He continued, "It would be surprising if we could, considering it is less than two hundred years since our European forebears were regarding a harsh and barren land with horror and despair. John White, principal surgeon of the First Fleet and of the colony of New South Wales, called the country a 'place so forbidding and so hateful as only to merit execrations and curses – a source of expense to the mother country and of evil and misfortune to its inhabitants.' Is there any link across perhaps a mere four or five generations between that view and our own?"

Medical histories of settlement have characterised many of the convicts as mentally ill. That would be unsurprising, given the desperation that often led to their crimes, their social isolation and the experience of a death sentence being imposed, then commuted to transportation for life to a place that may as well have been the moon.

Construction of the first purpose-built psychiatric facility in Australia, the Tarban Creek Lunatic Asylum in New South Wales, finished in 1838. Previously, mentally ill people were housed in the town gaol at Parramatta or the female factory or the former convict barracks of the abandoned government farm at Castle Hill, where the first doctors were convicts themselves and untrained attendants were selected for their size and strength.

The state of Victoria's mental hospitals are older than the state of Victoria. The first purpose-built institution opened in 1848 as a local ward of the Tarban Creek asylum. In 1851, it was renamed Yarra Bend Asylum. Above a sinuous trail where the waters of the Merri Creek meet those of the Yarra River, a bluestone building sat surrounded by a rolling landscape which none of its "inmates" could see. A year passed before reports leaked out. The ensuing parliamentary inquiry heard evidence about patients being sexually and physically abused, filthy facilities, corruption, misappropriation. A new administrator was installed, but conditions continued to deteriorate. There were 251 inmates by 1855; 450 by 1858. A proposal for a new mental hospital in Kew stalled in parliament. So Yarra Bend expanded, new wards built cheaply around the bluestone building, all of it always about to close, no use throwing good money after bad. By 1870, Yarra Bend housed over 1000 people. It operated for another fifty-five years.

"For some time back," a reader named "Humanitas" wrote to The Argus in 1874, "the bodies of patients who die in the Yarra Bend are buried by 'contract'; and the contractor is in the habit of conveying the dead bodies to the cemetery in an open spring cart, without a particle of clothing except a small bit of well-worn oil cloth." The letter continued:

> The effluvia from the cart is often something horrible, and to make the matter worse, the contractor is in the habit of driving along this road at the rate of about 10 miles an hour – portions of the road are rough patches of new metal etc.

"Rattle his bones over the stones,

He's only a looney whom nobody owns."

Surely this should not be allowed in this Christian land ...

Not even a century into settlement, there was a glaring gap between values and behaviour – between the offer of asylum and the reality. That gap remains.

*

As the fate of the institutionalised shows, mental illness in the colonies was deeply stigmatised, despite its prevalence. Stigma is a complex social process that excludes or devalues someone on the basis of a particular characteristic. At the time of the Fifth National Mental Health and Suicide Prevention Plan (2017), the stigma attached to mental illness was so prevalent in Australia that most of us had experienced it. The "ever-presence of stigma and dis-crimination" for those with mental illness – as the federal Select Committee on Mental Health and Suicide Prevention put it in 2021 – was identified as a major barrier to treatment and recovery by both the federal Productivity Commission in 2020 and the Royal Commission into Victoria's Mental Health System in 2021. Its impacts are compounded for those who experi-ence additional forms of discrimination, such as Aboriginal and Torres Strait Islander peoples and people who identify as LGBTIQ+.

The sociologist Erving Goffman elaborated his theory of stigma in a slim 1963 study, *Stigma: Notes on the Management of Spoiled Identity*. In his terms, the stigmatised individual is "deeply discredited" by society. They are demoted in their entitlement to social participation, and basic respect, because of a gap between their actual social identity (member of the diverse human race) and their virtual, or assigned, social identity (polluted, spoiled, threat, scapegoat). "We construct ... an ideology to explain his inferiority and account for the danger he represents," Goffman explained of the stig-matised individual. "We use specific stigma terms such as cripple, bastard, moron in our daily discourse as a source of metaphor and imagery, typically without giving thought to the original meaning." *Totally crazy, right? A complete psycho. Just madness. Absolutely manic. Schizo. Insane!*

In Goffman's taxonomy, the Normals are the counterpoint to the Stigmatised, policing proximity to society and its benefits. "While the stranger is present before us," Goffman wrote, "evidence can arise of his possessing an attribute that makes him different from others in the category of persons available for him to be, and of a less desirable kind – in the extreme, a person who is quite thoroughly bad, or dangerous, or weak. He is thus reduced in our minds from a whole and usual person to a tainted discounted one." This constellation of prejudicial, exclusionary and limiting beliefs manifests in social interactions, in healthcare, in mass media, in apparently neutral rules and procedures, and eventually it can invade the stigmatised person's inner life. For these reasons, stigma can both cause and exacerbate poor mental health.

No one wrote like Goffman, least of all in mid-century academia; his prose is jaunty and brutal and much of it now reads as outdated. But his incisiveness stands and it comes down to this: at its heart – and it is a hot human heart of animal muscle and accelerating blood – stigma is driven by a need for belonging, but its monstrous tactics ultimately condemn it to be self-defeating. This is because one of the lies Normals tell themselves concerns the universality of vulnerability. No moral charge attaches to something like a cold because of its prevalence and fleeting physical impact. However, despite also being prevalent and treatable, mental illness receives no such leeway. It is instead conflated with weakness, badness, wilfulness, something that only happens to others, something to be feared and, in effect, something to be punished. The question, then, is: why?

*

The mental health system in Australia was failing, even before the pandemic, to provide adequate treatment and support to those who need it. The Victorian Royal Commission comprehensively detailed what this looks like on the ground – and the picture is essentially the same throughout the nation, as demonstrated by the 2020 federal Productivity Commission's inquiry report on mental health.

Almost half of all Australian adults will experience mental ill-health during their lives, and almost one in five will meet the criteria in a given year. These numbers have likely risen during the pandemic. A 2019 survey carried out by the Australian Education Union indicated that 72 per cent of secondary teachers reported that self-harm had occurred in their schools in the past year. Victoria Police responded to a mental health call-out about every twelve minutes in 2017–18.

In 2018–19, approximately 3189 people presented at the Austin Health emergency department for mental health issues: that equates to at least one person arriving in extreme distress every three hours, continuously, for one year. That's one metropolitan public hospital. Even before Covid-19 hit, emergency departments were under-resourced to treat an unceasing stream of people who should have had better and earlier options for help.

In 2019–20, there were 3.3 million missing hours. That's the difference between what was required and the actual hours of community mental health treatment and support delivered by public services. It's an anaemic measure of unmet demand until you think about how long a minute is when you are desperate for help that does not come, and how one person's pain passes on to others.

Because of the continuing strength of the stigma attached to mental illness, most Australians do not seek help for symptoms either at all or until they have drastically deteriorated. However, there is no "us" and "them" when it comes to health; mental illness is something anyone can experience, not just Others. By drastically increasing calls to crisis lines and psychiatric admissions to emergency departments, especially for children, the pandemic has proved any basis for the stigma false; but will that be enough to eliminate it?

In this essay, you will encounter three people whose interactions with the state while at their most unwell made them sicker. You will see the stigma that attaches to mental illness, and to anyone constructed as Other, and you will encounter those at the frontlines of how this stigma plays out. Their experiences indicate that despite the rhetoric of care and equality, our public institutions have often operated to penalise vulnerability, and that they have done so with collective consent. But all that might be about to change. In February 2021, the Victorian Royal Commission delivered its final report. In response, the state government committed to act on its recommendations in full. It is the most significant commitment to operationalising change made by an Australian jurisdiction, and the prevailing mood in relation to these promises is optimistic. I've spent a year sifting through the evidence before the commissioners and speaking with stakeholders around the nation in an effort to understand what our odds are for deep change.

Because this is a story about the mental health system, it is also a story about housing and hospitals and policing and prisons; classrooms, courtrooms, bedrooms and waiting rooms. It is about what could happen when U too R not OK. It is not about money; it is about where we choose to spend money. It is about things that increase the risk of mental illness: isolation, trauma, stigma, socioeconomic disadvantage and genetics. It is about who gets a fair go and why. It is about siloes, mateship and connective tissue. And while we will talk about recovery and redemption, it is always about history.

"For too long mental health has been relegated to the shadows within the broader health system," stated the Victorian Royal Commission's 2019 interim report. "Many are left to exist on the margins; many feel unbearably alone and defeated when the right services are not available to them; and some take their own lives. There has been some progress, but stigma, discrimination and prejudice remain pervasive influences on the lives of people living with mental illness. As a community, we have struggled to understand mental illness and the varying ways people experience it. Some might say we have lacked the empathy to support people who are struggling." The sheer prevalence of mental illness indicates that this relegation of mental health "to the shadows" is not only a lack of empathy – it's also a lack of self-compassion. This in turn indicates it has something to do with fear and shame.

In the analytical psychology of Carl Jung, we have both a conscious persona and a Shadow. Our Shadow contains the hidden parts of ourselves we are taught to revile. In a healthy psyche, these different parts are integrated. But where early life events have had an unaddressed impact, those parts are likely to be unconsciously dissociated, consigned to the depths. And they are more prone to the process of projection, in which our own "faults" – the thing we have no wish to be, as Jung put it – are experienced only as someone else's failings. Jung saw that if the contents of the Shadow remain unexplored and unintegrated, they will be at the root of problems between individuals and within groups, fuelling prejudice and sparking conflicts.

On the other hand, recognition of the Shadow, as he wrote in *Civilisation in Transition*, is a connecting force. "A human relationship is not based on differentiation and perfection, for these only emphasize the differences or call forth the exact opposite; it is based rather on imperfection, on what is weak, helpless and in need of support – the very ground and motive for dependence." We lose much – personally and collectively – by remaining perniciously incurious about what is kept in the darkest, oldest rooms of ourselves.

*

This is not to say that we aren't moved to attempt to find solutions. Announcing his state's royal commission in February 2019, Premier Daniel Andrews said that the mental health system was broken. Over the next two years, the commissioners tried to hit a moving target – mapping the landscape of a system that was failing disastrously before the onset of the pandemic. The submissions made clear that people do not know how or where to seek help for mental illness. That they do not, and frequently cannot, access help until they are in extreme distress. That aside from being severely understaffed and under-resourced, services are siloed – incapable of effective communication or cooperation. In the commission's final report, the phrases "service gap" and "service gaps" appear 104 times. Those gaps, and the knowledge that marginalised people fall through them, are not new; they are mentioned in reports on dysfunction in the mental healthcare systems of every state and territory, and have been for decades. One could drown in the grey literature generated since the first National Mental Health Plan in 1993. What those thousands of pages indicate is that the gaps are not limited to the sterile administrative realm of "services." The disconnection runs deeper; it appears to be embodied.

The commission's recommendations "centred on transformational reform." The goal: "to rebalance the system so that more services will be delivered in community settings, and extend beyond a health response to a more holistic approach to good mental health and wellbeing across the community." The promised change is monumental, from the official acknowledgment that "mental health is shaped by the social, cultural, economic and physical environments in which people live and is a shared responsibility of society," to the government's full commitment to the report's recommendations at a cost of $3.8 billion. The reforms envisage a mental health and wellbeing system "for all."

While the vision is new, promises are not. If you are passingly familiar with the history of public inquiries into mental healthcare in Australia, the mission of the latest Victorian royal commission may have evoked a strange déjà vu. "Inquiries are not new in mental health," Professor Ian Hickie and

Sebastian Rosenberg wrote in *The Conversation* in 2018. "There were 32 separate statutory inquiries into the sector between 2006 and 2012 alone." They noted that "very few, if any" of the recommendations had been implemented. In 2018, there were "no fewer than 14 inquiries or independent reviews." This was "business as usual" for the mental health sector, Jennifer Doggett wrote in *Inside Story* that year. "Despite numerous past inquiries and reviews of various aspects of the mental health system," the Productivity Commission reported in 2020, "there remains considerable need and scope for reform." On page 1088 of its report, it noted that the then-current National Mental Health Strategy comprised seven documents totalling over 300 pages. "Insofar as it retains priorities of past plans it risks everything becoming a priority and little being fully accomplished."

Since 1854, the state has held royal commissions into, among other things: sludge removal (1858), defence (1858), cattle disease (1863), prison discipline (1870), diphtheria (1872), policing (1881, 1905), taxes (1881), butter (1904) and sewerage (1925). There have been more royal commissions concerning vegetables (1885, 1915) than for Indigenous communities (1877). More royal commissions concerning world fairs (1861, 1878, 1889, 1890) than for mental healthcare (1884, 1924, 2021). Royal or otherwise, commissions and public inquiries are a longstanding institutional feature of politics in Australia. They are used to serve a specialised fact-finding and/or advisory function. Another function: they buy time by providing the optics of accountability where an issue has got out of hand or is incapable of a satisfactorily popular fix. A 2011 report by the Victorian Parliamentary Research Service noted it is unclear where royal commissions fit into the accountability mechanisms of the political and legal systems. This might be their appeal.

Since the Royal Commission into Aboriginal Deaths in Custody ended in 1991, there have been over 500 Aboriginal deaths in custody. Since the Royal Commission into Family Violence ended in 2015, intimate partner homicide has remained the most common form of homicide in Australia and most victims are women. Since the Royal Commission into

Institutional Responses to Child Sexual Abuse, the processes of the National Redress Scheme have been found to be traumatising for survivors. Since the Royal Commission into Aged Care Quality and Safety, lack of expertise and preparedness in aged-care facilities has resulted in large-scale failures to manage Covid-19, with fatal consequences. Public inquiries are a ritual of Australian society through which the violated moral order is condemned and an idealised image of the collective is restored. However, our lack of loyalty to their findings indicates that, as an electorate, we value optics over operationalisation.

So too for mental healthcare reform. Despite the fact that "there are few, if any, areas of government activity more formally examined than mental health services and suicide prevention" – as Mental Health Australia noted in 2021 – regardless of what Australian jurisdiction you currently find yourself in, the mental healthcare system will be in crisis. It appears to be our habit to invest attention only so far and no further, and then to do it again and again. By this point, that impulse towards repetition appears compulsive.

We may say, Sigmund Freud wrote, about the repetition compulsion he had observed in his practice, "that the patient does not *remember* anything of what he has forgotten and repressed, but *acts* it out. He reproduces it not as memory but as an action; he *repeats* it, without, of course, knowing that he is repeating it."

*

All of this activity runs up against something, but what? What social structure, what forgetting, what fear, what shame? Perhaps, when it comes to this "sickness unprevented for all our diligence," to use the 400-year-old words of John Donne, we will have to look elsewhere for change, towards something "unsuspected for all our curiositie."

First used by Freud in his 1894 paper "The Neuro-Psychoses of Defence," the term "defence mechanism" would come to describe the group of predominantly unconscious mental processes we all rely on to reach palatable solutions to painful interior conflicts we are unable or unwilling to resolve. These defences shield us from suffering threats to our preferred self-concept, so in that limited sense they are adaptive.

For example, we block out uncomfortable ideas, experiences and drives (repression). We displace our unwanted feelings onto others, where they continue to menace us but from a safer distance (projection). We refuse to integrate the existence of painful facts (denial). We seek safe, but false, explanations (rationalisation). To a certain extent, this is all a normal part of mental functioning. Defence mechanisms become pathological, however, through excessive or rigid use, at which point "respect for reality," as Freud put it elsewhere, is lost and significant harm can be caused to ourselves and others.

Splitting is another common defence mechanism. At its most general, splitting is a form of psychological dismemberment following a failure to reconcile the inevitable positive and negative qualities of ourselves or others into a coherent, realistically human whole. It involves splitting off certain repellent characteristics from ourselves, or others, to create an artificial image which only creates more instability and pain.

The Australian settlement was built on two enormous acts of splitting: transportation and terra nullius. The public institutions we routinely invest with power whenever we vote originated on stolen land amid one of the most marginalised sections of the British population and those who sought to build wealth off their backs. In important ways, those groups remain with us; their pain and their drives continue to haunt the body (and psyche) politic.

The colony's first collective sense of itself was one of precarity and scarcity; a spark flickering in a void. In early 1790, the NSW settlers were existing at "a bare subsistence level." Soon, arrivals at Sydney Cove were greeted by the "bloody sight of corpses rotting from swinging gibbets on the harbour." Seemingly the opposite of the prisons and hulks of Britain, the open penal settlements retained the defining power dynamic of those closed environments where perceived weakness invited violence.

In his 2019 study of madness in the colony, *Bedlam at Botany Bay*, James Dunk writes that "even if they avoided the worst of convict discipline, [the convicts] still lived in the fickle grip of masters, overseers, magistrates and governors, while the empire worked its policies out. The empire sought and achieved terror." State-sanctioned violence is a sloppy regulatory tool because its permissions spread. "Free colonists found that they were not safe from the power the government wielded against convicts. This power was the cause of much tension in the early decades of the colonial presence."

In the burgeoning colony — "where discipline, security and industry were fundamental to the business of a fragile government" — new opportunities for agency and earning unavailable to their counterparts in Britain were presented as the other side of the traumas experienced by convicts and free men. But "if we slow down," Dunk advises, "and listen closely, we find that doubt, anxiety, grief, and despair intrude into [the] familiar stories."

"Little of the colony's madness was attributed at the time to the violence of colonisation," Dunk notes. "Nevertheless, we are painfully conscious of the ways that warfare and other forms of savagery typically etch their brutal stories in hidden places." From 1794, there were at least 270 frontier massacres over 140 years as part of an increasingly lethal, state-sanctioned attempt to eradicate Aboriginal people. Bodies were disposed of in different ways, usually to conceal the massacre. "The stories of 'the killing times' are the ones we have heard in secret, or told in hushed tones," wrote Lorena Allam and Nick Evershed in *The Guardian* in 2019. "They are not the stories that appear in our history books yet they refuse to go away."

*

During the first fifty years of British settlement in Australia, the dominant demographic was white and male: a populace divided by factors so flimsy they required a brutal vigilance. We talk about tall poppies, but in the inchoate social environment of the carceral colony short poppies didn't stand a chance. This is part of our living inheritance. *She'll be right. Pretty ordinary. Toughen up.* A self-defeating disavowal of our own vulnerability thinly disguised as a lack of tolerance or responsibility for the pain of others.

In the settler population, there remained more men than women well into the twentieth century. "According to traditional gender norms, men should be self-reliant, assertive, competitive, violent when needed, and in control of their emotions," wrote Pauline Grosjean, professor of economics at UNSW, in *The Conversation* in 2021. Using data from Australia's "convict past," Grosjean, Victoria Baranov and Ralph De Haas found that "those early days of intensified competition between men [for female partners], and the violence that stemmed from this, created behaviours – and dangerous norms about masculinity – that continue in modern Australia today."

"We used historical census data and combined them with current data on violence, sexual and domestic assault, suicide and bullying in schools," Grosjean reported, explaining how they found that convict settlement areas in New South Wales, the Australian Capital Territory and Tasmania which had significantly more men than women in their first years still experience higher rates of these problems today. This remained true even accounting for present-day education, religion, urbanisation and income levels. In these areas, there is an otherwise-unexplained high share of men choosing stereotypically male occupations. People were less likely to support same-sex marriage. The data on health outcomes was also interesting. "Evidence suggests men adhering to traditional masculinity norms have a stronger stigma around mental health problems and tend to avoid health services. We found areas that were more historically male have significantly higher rates of male suicide today."

*

Australian historical orthodoxy has it that we eventually conquered the tyranny of distance and isolation – that we've "risen above our brutal beginnings," as Prime Minister Scott Morrison put it in his 2021 Australia Day speech. But we haven't truly started. Though we are not the only country struggling to reduce the incidence of suicide, Australia's suicide rate is higher than that of the United Kingdom, New Zealand and Canada. In her 2018 *Inside Story* article, Doggett noted that, in 1992, suicide accounted for 1.9 per cent of total deaths in Australia. "That was before the national mental health strategy and national depression initiative, and when barely anyone had heard of Prozac," she wrote. "Twenty-five years (and five national mental health plans) later, with Medicare payments for mental health services at $22 million a week and almost a tenth of the population taking antidepressants, suicides still make up 1.9 per cent of deaths." The most recent data shows that suicide continues to account for 1.9 per cent of deaths.

The aptly named General Record of Incidence of Mortality (GRIM) books are Excel spreadsheets of data collated by the Australian Institute of Health and Welfare on causes of death. Suicide is classified under "Injury: Intentional self-harm." In 2018, suicide was the leading cause of death among Australian children and adolescents. Greater than the road toll, it was also the leading cause of death for Australians between fifteen and forty-four. Men aged eighty-five and over had the highest age-specific rate of suicide, females aged forty to forty-four had the second-highest. While the causes of suicide are complex, and suicide remains difficult to predict, an Orygen report found that mental ill-health was present in around 90 per cent of young people who died by suicide. Other risk factors include trauma, abuse, discrimination, addiction and economic insecurity.

The suicide rate in the Indigenous population is double that of the non-Indigenous population, with the highest child suicide and female suicide rate in the country. LGBTIQ+ young people aged sixteen to seventeen are five times more likely to have attempted suicide than the rest of the general population; trans young people between sixteen and twenty-five are fifteen times more likely. Rates of self-harm among asylum seekers in Australia are "exceptionally high," with rates highest in immigration detention. People in rural areas are twice as likely to die by suicide. Given the exacerbating impacts of Covid-19, mental healthcare reform is more necessary now than ever before. And, like I said, the prevailing mood is optimistic. But that optimism might be misplaced, given there are few things as persistent as the patterns of the unaddressed past in the present.

Despite our willingness to connect sunnier characterisations of the "national character" to our national history, there is a conspicuous reluctance to explore the darker aspects through that same lens. And yet 125 years of psychoanalysis has demonstrated that – when it comes to human behaviour – extraordinary injuries can give rise to extraordinary defences. The body politic cannot fit in a therapist's room. Perhaps, however, we would gain insight by transposing the knowledge accumulated there about human actions and reactions onto our enduring collective behavioural patterns. It's a suggestive framework for understanding the water we swim in. This is where my mind goes when I hear the stories in the following chapters of people adrift in the colony, or drowning.

One wall of the conference room in Berry Street's Richmond office is a window. Through the glass pours a diffuse light that coats the white walls, the dark carpet, the surface of the table, the fidget spinners on it, and the 21-year-old hand silently causing one of those gadgets to rotate speedily. This hand belongs to a young woman I will call Eliza, who is telling me about her work as a lived experience consultant for Berry Street's Y-Change initiative, a role she has held for the past four years. To understand how remarkable it is that Eliza is sitting in this room making time to talk to me about her work, you must first understand a few things. She has survived childhood sexual abuse, physical abuse, psychological abuse and homelessness. She was expelled from school in Year 8. She's had four hospital admissions for acute distress and suicidal ideation. And she manages borderline personality disorder (BPD), which means dealing not only with symptoms which range from the inconvenient to the life-constricting, but also with the stigma that attends this diagnosis.

Our personalities are signature ways of thinking, feeling and behaving that distinguish us from others. Personality disorder is a complex and severe mental disorder estimated to affect approximately 6 per cent of the global population. According to the American Psychiatric Association's *Diagnostic and Statistical Manual of Mental Disorders*, it is an enduring way of thinking, feeling and behaving that deviates from socio-cultural norms, causes distress or problems functioning.

The DSM's categorical approach specifies ten types of personality disorder, which one can be diagnosed as having singly or in combination. Whether that diagnosis identifies antisocial personality disorder or the avoidant, borderline, dependant, histrionic, narcissistic, obsessive-compulsive, paranoid, schizoid or schizotypal type, each involves a persistent, pervasive pattern that begins around late adolescence or early adulthood and impairs at least two of the following areas: how one thinks about oneself and others; how one relates to others; emotional responses;

and behavioural regulation. An alternative diagnostic model, adopted by the World Health Organization, is more concerned with functional impact than discrete typologies. Whichever lens is chosen, it remains true that personality disorder is enduring and can be severely impairing, similar in these respects to intellectual disability and autism spectrum disorders.

Personality disorders were long considered untreatable. That is no longer the case. While treatment type depends on individual circumstances, psychotherapy – sometimes with medication – is currently considered the best way of gaining insight and learning coping techniques. In the frosty language of public health, although personality disorder is associated with high service usage and treatment costs, the economic benefits of evidence-based therapeutic intervention have been established. Which is to say, recovery is achievable. However, personality disorder has received minimal recognition as a public health issue. Until very recently, for example, its incidence was not tracked by the Australian Institute of Health and Welfare. Untreated individuals may be unable to learn or work, they can develop additional mental health issues such as drug or alcohol addiction, they may fall into social disadvantage and they also have a high suicide risk. The impact spreads. One clinician I speak with says that, in their experience, division among staff in relation to a patient can indicate the presence of BPD. "In view of the substantially increased stress levels seen in family members of individuals with BPD, and the increased risk of developing BPD among children of mothers with the condition, targeted interventions for these groups need to be developed and evaluated," a recent article in The Lancet stated.

BPD is characterised by a pervasive pattern of emotional dysregulation, including impulsivity; unstable and inconsistent identity; and problems in interpersonal relations. Someone with BPD "may go to great lengths to avoid being abandoned, have repeated suicide attempts, display inappropriate intense anger or have ongoing feelings of emptiness," states the American Psychiatric Association. Those with BPD tend to displace their own unacceptable feelings or impulses onto others at a greater level of intensity. They tend to express contradictory feelings or beliefs, without being concerned by the inconsistency. They tend to idealise others in unrealistic ways, followed by swift devaluation and attack. They will often experience an inability to settle into life roles (education, work, relationships) due to this emotional lability, unstable self-image and difficulty with affect regulation. Sufferers have high rates of self-harming behaviours and substance abuse.

Although BPD is a serious mental disorder and its symptoms can improve with treatment, there is a general belief, which is also not uncommon among those who work in mental health, that those with the diagnosis are immoral (in the sense of being deliberately manipulative or dangerous), beyond help or hope. Doctors have spoken to me of a prevalent therapeutic nihilism. A mental health researcher told me that patients with the diagnosis have been deprioritised on hospital wards. A peer support worker once advised Eliza not to tell her new psychologist that she had been diagnosed with BPD. "The diagnosis of BPD has few friends," wrote Dr Andrew Chanen, director of clinical services at Orygen, in *Australasian Psychiatry*.

"It is the only disorder, I would argue, in all of health, that you can get away with saying things about a patient that no one else would dare say," Chanen told me. "Having been around in the era when 'schizophrenia' was a dirty word, or when 'HIV' was a dirty word, people said awful things about those patients. Now you would never hear anybody say those things, yet it is still seen as acceptable to say the most disgraceful, bigoted things about individuals with BPD, and to see their behaviour as wilful."

*

Eliza lives with her cat in an inner-city apartment she moved to from an outer suburb of Melbourne. She enjoys scrapbooking and, like me, cried watching the Disney movie *Luca*, because it so movingly portrays the process of shedding shame. She does not have frequent contact with her father. She speaks with compassion for her mother, a single parent who struggled with financial stress, housing insecurity, addiction, and physical domestic violence as well as coercive control while raising Eliza and her siblings. Remaining at home was not in Eliza's best interest, but there was great pressure to stay. One of Eliza's greatest fears is that she will be responsible – because of something she has done or, more accurately, because of who she is – for her utter abandonment by loved ones. A need to release the intense distress of this feeling has previously led her to significant self-harm. Given this, the natural act of individuation required to leave home to work near the city was akin to scaling an alp. She did it anyway because of something in her character which has survived like those microbes that thousands of years of frost cannot kill. This something is separate from her disorder, her personality structure and the limiting beliefs implanted in her as a result of her traumatic childhood; it may be accurate to call this something Eliza's Self.

On a number of occasions, over our time talking together, I feel I have seen something of this essential character. It is in her integrity (times when she has chosen being right over being liked), her bravery (times when she has spoken frankly about experiences she admits cause her shame), her persistence despite extreme adversity, her life-embracing curiosity and her intelligence (despite having internalised the belief that she is "not good at school," she speaks fluently in a professional and emotional vocabulary it took me – with many years of tertiary education – much longer to grasp).

Eliza is an outlier: literally extraordinary. People living with complex mental illness are more likely than the general population to die by suicide. For Australians living with schizophrenia, the risk is thirteen times greater; for those living with bipolar disorder, seventeen times greater; for those with major depressive disorder, twenty times greater; and for those with BPD, the risk is forty-five times greater. Moreover, of the 174 young people in custody in Victoria's Youth Justice Centres in the year 2018–19, 67 per cent had been victims of abuse, trauma or neglect, 68 per cent had been suspended or expelled from school, 54 per cent had a history of both drug and alcohol misuse, 35 per cent had been the subject of a child protection order, 48 per cent presented with mental health issues and 27 per cent had a history of self-harm or suicidal thoughts. Statistically, she should be there, but she is here, calming herself by turning the fidget spinner on a broad, clean table.

"I never, ever, ever in my wildest dreams *ever* thought I would live to eighteen," she says. "I didn't think about what I wanted to be when I grew up because I knew I wasn't gonna be there. When I got to seventeen and was about to turn eighteen, I was really lost and wasn't expecting to be there."

Though we are sitting in a sleek, modern office, Berry Street was founded in 1877 as the Victorian Infant Asylum to support single mothers and their children. It is now one of Australia's largest independent family service organisations. Its programs include support for family violence, education, trauma, parenting and out-of-home care. The Y-Change team trains and employs young people with personal experience of socio-economic disadvantage to act as lived experience consultants – advising government and a range of organisations on the design and delivery of social services.

"Young people at Y-Change have been forced to carry the systemic trauma of systems that have failed them," explains Morgan Cataldo, who leads the team. "We seek to break up that power dynamic by investing in young people long-term, ensuring that their lived expertise is at the heart of informing how we think and act." One of the reasons for optimism following the Royal Commission is the new awareness shown by the current government that those with personal experience of the mental health system will often have the most valuable reflections of how the system is failing.

Eliza entered the mental health system at twelve, when school friends saw she'd been self-harming and told a teacher, who sent her to the school counsellor. "I think, in a way, I was asking for help," she says. Though initially uncomfortable speaking with the male counsellor, she gradually opened up enough to share that she was having suicidal thoughts; that she "didn't want to be here anymore." Nearly a decade later, she says this quickly, the words melding and her voice receding under the weight of it. Without informing Eliza, the counsellor called her mother, who reacted strongly. "That was kind of like getting punished for talking about what's going on," Eliza explains. "I was like, 'I'm never fucking talking to anyone anymore because when you do, you get into trouble.' I started to know I had to hide it better." Now she understands her mother's reaction as a mix of love and fear in a single parent who had herself been struggling. "It was a really big shock to Mum. Because she'd dealt with it in her family." Close relatives had been diagnosed with bipolar disorder, and one had killed themself. Diagnosed with depression, Eliza was given a herbal supplement by her mother that she refers to now as "the sad powder" with a distancing laugh. Two years later, she would be hospitalised for suicidal ideation.

"When I was fourteen, I didn't know at the time but I was experiencing family violence and homelessness," she explains, about the water she then swam in. "And also a recent sexual assault." She started drinking daily, doing drugs, spending time in places where that was the norm. At school, she was regularly sent out of class for being disruptive or for not wearing the correct uniform, which was not achievable because she did not own a complete uniform and the items she had were not in good condition. One teacher she remembers fondly. She would sit in the quiet of his office after being kicked out of class. He would give her face wipes when she broke the rule about wearing make-up, and canteen vouchers when she had no food or money. He bought her tights to wear in winter and helped with her assignments. "He was really good," she says, "but the person above him, the coordinator for the year level, was like, 'She has to go.' Which I do understand, because there was a fight at school. But I did apologise." She fought with another student. "I threw a chair at a teacher. I stole some food. And I got expelled after that," she explains, resigned. "They asked me to leave, but they didn't tell me where to go. They just said I wasn't allowed to come within a certain amount of feet of the schoolgrounds."

"At the time I got excluded from school – expelled – I'd been struggling with mental health since I was twelve. So though Years 7 and 8, I was really struggling and school wasn't ..." She trails off and is silent for a moment, during which blood blooms beneath the surface of her cheeks.

"First of all, it wasn't for me. I couldn't learn, I couldn't sit still. I was the destructive kid. And I would come to school with self-harm scars then get sent home because they were like, 'We don't know what the fuck to do, you need to go home.' Which was even more isolating and it made me feel worse. I didn't feel like school was a safe place for me."

I look at the car park through the window that is a wall, imagining Eliza at fourteen; it's not hard, her face is still so young. I think about what teachers are taught about difficult behaviour. And the devastating consequences of mistaking the last note for the whole song. "Looking back," Eliza continues, "even if they'd asked me, I wouldn't have been able to tell them, because I didn't know what I'd been through, at first. And I didn't know how to tell them."

Referring to the period known as childhood, she says, "It was a very violent situation but I don't remember much 'cause I was a kid." Eliza was very young when her parents separated, and while that solved some problems, new ones arose. "We were homeless with Mum," she says, explaining that for a time, they lived in a tent. "Mum told me we were having a holiday. It took me a while to realise; I guess you don't know what you don't know."

The Productivity Commission report found that one-quarter of all people admitted to acute mental health services are homeless prior to admission and most are discharged back into homelessness. Victoria has the lowest provision of social housing in the country. Although priority is given to those on low incomes who have experienced homelessness, family violence or mental illness, over 100,000 people are waitlisted for housing. A quarter of the state's homeless population are aged between twelve and twenty-four; 6000 young people have no safe place to sleep each night. Many of them are homeless due to family violence. This is not new. Following decades of underinvestment, the Victorian government is investing $5.3 billion – the biggest single spend on social and affordable housing in the state's history – to build over 12,000 homes within four years. Two thousand of the homes will be allocated to people with mental illness. In

2021, Melbourne City Mission and the Salvation Army called on the government to also reserve a proportion of the homes for young people.

"Mum was working full-time, trying to afford for us kids. She was always working," Eliza says. Much of the time she was alone with her siblings. The family eventually moved to a hotel, then to a house. Although they finally had a home, it wasn't large enough for the children to have their own rooms, and Eliza was scared of an older male relative who spent time in the house. When she describes the impact of his behaviour on her and her youngest sibling, it is with a deep understanding of intergenerational trauma, how it is held in a body and moves through a psyche. Her cheeks redden again, and she needs to take a break. It is a false strength that cannot ask for help or rest; that is the kind of pretence that serves a function in closed or dangerous environments. *She'll be right.* By refusing to play into that illusion, Eliza is modelling something enormously important and that is why I am telling you now.

Her memories of getting Littlest Pet Shop toys for Christmas exist alongside memories of being chased through her home by someone with a knife, knowing there was no one to call for help. One of the reasons relational trauma can be harder to resile from than physical trauma is the element of confusion introduced into the young mind when instances of warmth and love exist alongside instances of abuse or emotional abandonment. In that situation, a child will make sense of abuse by pinning blame on themselves and unconsciously forbidding any knowledge of justified anger towards the parent in order to preserve the possibility of the protector's grand return. It is, at first, an adaptive survival strategy, but eventually that form of dissociation becomes torturous and life-constricting.

"I didn't know what to call it, but it felt wrong," Eliza says. "I tried to tell the teacher, but they didn't understand the full extent of it and I probably didn't say it very well." After her expulsion at fourteen, she had "a difficult time." She was misdiagnosed with depression and put on antidepressants. She initially attended a mental health program for children not in school, but her self-harming escalated until her mother locked away everything sharp in the house. If she needed scissors for scrapbooking, she had to wait for her mum to get home. Her mother was overwhelmed, struggling with addiction. An attempt at living with her father was disastrous, resulting in Eliza taking out an intervention order against him. She started running away, consequently missing her appointments with the psychologist. She became homeless.

Despite the intervention order, her father would file missing person reports and the police would track her down, throw her in a divvy van and drop her back at his place. "They treated me like a criminal." These were months of sleeping in dark places with empty refrigerators, where a child wouldn't think twice about adults racking lines on their phone screen. The idea of becoming a mum at fourteen seemed alluring – not for the Centrelink money, as those around her advised, but to have someone to love and to love her. "And then there was my first admission, which, looking back, makes sense, but at the time it was really confusing. I felt like they just saw the surface level – 'Oh, she's self-harming, we need to stop those behaviours' – without actually understanding why things were really hard for me.

"For hours, hours, I waited in the waiting room and I was lucky that first time to get a bed," she explains. "The first time was really scary. I didn't really know what was going on or what was going to happen." After she was released, the children's mental health program she had attended referred her to a mobile psychologist. "He would meet me at the library, or he'd come to Mum's." Eliza shared some things with him, but was not yet able to verbalise the trauma she had experienced.

At fifteen, she decided to stop seeing that psychologist. Only when she saw the discharge paper addressed to her mother did she learn he had diagnosed her with BPD. Like the earlier depression diagnosis, her mother had dismissed it. Eliza thinks that perhaps her mother was in denial, maybe worried about the stigma that would adversely affect her daughter. She is, however, angry with the clinical decision not to inform her about her own health. "That's another problem in the mental health system, but also in surrounding systems – they don't talk to children and young people."

After the children's mental health program ended, she started working at McDonald's. The near-impossibility of working through her bad days made her believe, at seventeen, that she would always be incapable of holding a job. The work environment was unaccommodating of physical illness, so she learnt to conceal her mental illness, even immediately following her next hospital admission. She was placed in a small psychiatric assessment and planning unit, located next to the emergency department, which provided short-term, specialised emergency mental healthcare. Eliza explains that because it only had four beds, "you're very lucky to get a spot." After being discharged, she maintained some contact with area mental health services. But, ultimately, she was a child who came to her own rescue.

After learning that some friends were attending classes at a flexi school (described as a space "outside conventional education" that addresses "the needs of disenfranchised young people"), Eliza went along one day and returned the next. She kept returning. This is how she earned her adult certificate of education, the equivalent of Year 10, which enabled her to enrol in Year 11 at a school that offered further educational qualifications. "I got myself into that," she says, proudly. "No person told me. I didn't even know flexi schools existed.

"I was seventeen, still having these issues, they weren't going away," she continues. At the alternative school she was attending, students could access free psychological and psychiatric services. She saw a psychiatrist and was diagnosed again with BPD. This time, however, she was given a detailed explanation of the diagnosis. "I was like, 'That makes so much fucking sense,'" she laughs, explaining what a relief it was to understand why she struggled with certain things and to discover that she wasn't being negative or dramatic or difficult or disruptive or sensitive or overemotional or ungrateful or a trouble maker or a bitch or a little shit. And that she wasn't alone.

*

Later, I'm walking and listening to a podcast in which three Jungian analysts discuss borderline personality disorder. One of them, Joseph Lee, explains that early in his career, "My supervisor said, 'I just want to give you a sense of how these borderline individuals probably feel, at least by the time they get here in the hospital.' Just imagine that you're four years old and you're walking onto a subway platform with your mum. You're holding hands. It's crowded, there's teeming people all around. The subway car pulls up. There's a huge rush of people and your mum loses contact with your hand and then in the next moment, the train begins to pull away and you see that your mum is in the subway car that's pulling out of the station. Imagine how that feels. And then imagine that most of the borderline disordered clients are feeling that most of every day."

Lee's deep voice is so gentle but the feeling he describes plunges into me like a fist, pulling the breath from my lungs in the middle of the footpath. When that feeling hits me – and it is not unfamiliar due to a relational trauma in my own life – I steady myself by looking at the sky, the tops of trees. Except that today when I do so, I think of Eliza, how strong she has been, and then, strangely, of aerophytes, those plants that thrive only on rain and air.

*

When Eliza describes what would have helped when she needed it most, her answer is both startling and not. The first thing would be housing and financial support for her mother. Then, having someone to talk to who understood how a child thinks about things too unsafe for them to understand, someone who could identify warning signs and connect her to services. Someone to support you, she explains, drive you to appointments and to school, take you driving or out for a coffee, ask how you're going. Someone who cares about what's happening in your life. Our systems are really confusing to navigate, she continues, explaining how she broke down in tears at Centrelink. They don't make any sense; young people shouldn't have to do everything by themselves. The surprise in what she says is due to what she is describing: the pre-existing roles of society's adult caregivers: parent, teacher, doctor.

Eliza applied for the role at Y-Change after seeing an ad on Facebook. "It talked about someone who had been through a lot and wanting to be a leader. I didn't think that I was capable of doing anything like that. But I applied anyway," she says, with a small laugh. She was successful in her interview. "I didn't expect ever to have a job that paid $25 an hour, so I was like, 'I don't deserve to be here at all.'"

Eliza had not yet disclosed the traumatic events she had experienced. "It was still looking at that surface level instead of getting to the root," she explains. She had started to discuss what she'd been through with a new psychologist, but felt betrayed when they called child services without informing her first. She felt without control or choice; that the psychologist didn't fully understand the situation. And, perhaps most significantly, that she'd been placed yet again in the eviscerating position of having to choose between being well and being loyal.

"All throughout that time, I was like, 'Oh, this is my fault.' Because that's what everyone told me. So I internalised that. Then, when I came here, I understood my family should've behaved differently, the school should've done more, the mental health service should've done it differently ... Y-Change helped me to understand that it wasn't my fault what I'd been through, and, instead of me constantly hating myself, it helped me to change perspective and see, 'Where were people in your life that are paid to be there and notice things for children to keep them safe, where did they fail you? And where did those systems fail you?'"

Many child victims of sexual assault who share their experience at the time of the abuse are not listened to: "we have almost an inherent blindness to it," Hayley Foster, CEO at Full Stop Australia (previously called Rape and Domestic Violence Services Australia), told *The Sydney Morning Herald*. Something that compounds trauma is being blamed for it – being made to carry the shame of others. When Eliza once said to me, "On paper, I would've looked like a really bad kid with my criminal record, doing drugs, not engaging with services, not engaged in school, not doing any-thing young people should be doing," my mind went to an image of a chair suspended between her outstretched fourteen-year-old arms and the body of a teacher. I wondered what it means to have a duty of care for children in a country where one in six women and one in nine men have experienced physical and/or sexual abuse before the age of fifteen? What prevents us investing properly in teacher training and support, given that reality? How many school employees does it take to approve an expulsion? What might it look like to hold space for the raging projections of a trau-matised child? I thought about how a wall can actually be a window. And it seemed then that Eliza was not the worst one when it came to a dysreg-ulated relationship to emotion.

*

The purpose of acute inpatient services in general hospitals is to sup-port those who cannot be effectively or safely treated in the community. However, the federal Productivity Commission found that, while not all hospitalisations are avoidable, "gaps in non-acute services in communi-ties lead to avoidable hospital admissions." Nationally, the rate of mental health presentations at emergency departments has risen by about 70 per cent over the past fifteen years, particularly due to lack of alternatives during evenings and weekends. For years, emergency departments have been left overwhelmed and under-resourced for the task, torn between the challenge of managing bed demand for incoming patients and that of safely discharging patients. Like those it exists to serve, the healthcare sys-tem required earlier intervention. Now, as I write this, psychiatric wards at Melbourne's major hospitals are being forced to close beds amid staff shortages caused by the Omicron wave.

The last time Eliza was admitted to hospital, she was eighteen. It required an enormous act of persistence when she was at her lowest. So it's easy to see how it might have gone differently, and I would be here speaking with someone else. She presented at the emergency department of a metropolitan hospital because she knew she could not keep herself "safe," by which she means alive. No beds were available. "You just have to wait for ages," she says, "even if you have physical self-harm scars. There's a person who's dying – they need support first, which is why it's hard that mental health has been so integrated into physical health. Because of that, [it] gets triaged last." She was told she could sleep, if necessary, in the waiting area, or go home. While that scenario feels particularly unsafe for survivors of sexual assault, she explains, nobody in crisis should have to sleep in a public waiting room. "And it's like, if I go home, I'm not safe: that's why I'm here.

"They gave me a Valium, but at the end of the day I was needing help and I got turned away. They said, 'You can come back tomorrow.' I came back and there was no beds. Came back the next day and there was no beds. I saw my psychologist every day that I was trying to get into the psych ward, so she could make sure I was still alive." Finally, a bed became available and she was admitted to the adult inpatient unit. "There's old men – which because of my previous experiences, and just in general, I didn't feel comfortable. They were making comments about my body, so that was a really unsafe situation." A nurse moved her to a gender-sensitive area of the ward. "But you still had to go out into the main room if you wanted to eat. So, it still wasn't safe for me and I was trying to focus on my recovery. There needs to be somewhere for young people to go, because it doesn't make sense. In what other system would you have eighteen-year-old [females] with sixty-year-old males? You don't do that in the prison systems – why is that in the mental health system?"

The Victorian Department of Health sums up the ideal functioning of acute inpatient services this way: they "provide a range of therapeutic interventions and programs to patients and their families to learn more about the impact of the illness, explore ways to better manage the illness, improve coping strategies and move towards recovery." This did not reflect Eliza's experience. She felt that she had insufficient time with the doctors. "They're always walking really fast 'cause they don't want to talk to patients.

No one really has time for you." The nurses' area was glass-shielded. "So it's almost like a prison – they're separated from you. If you want to talk to them, you have to knock on the glass. Sometimes they would ignore you. I do understand that the doctors and nurses are stretched for their time, but at the same time – we're there because we need support, and this is in a public mental health hospital."

She felt unaided in improving her coping strategies and moving towards recovery. "Imagine all these white walls, there's these massive lights," she says, explaining that there was nothing to do. Just TV. "The coloured pencils are all blunt because you're not allowed sharpeners. A small thing like being able to colour in would have made a big difference, but yeah …" she says, trailing off. "There was no therapeutic aspect to it, it was just like a holding cell until they kicked you out and the next person came in."

The feeling of being turned away while suicidal was familiar. She had felt it at home, and at school, after being honest about her needs.

"A lot of the problems associated with BPD are not part of the diagnostic criteria," Dr Chanen, at Orygen, had told me. "They're things that we create. Often people will take recurrent presentations to EDs, fights with the staff there, restraint and sedation and some of the more cruel practices as being diagnostic of BPD, whereas in fact they're diagnostic of the mental health system."

*

In Aristotelian terms, telos refers to something's inherent purpose or potential. A teleological view of history holds that we're always improving, only getting better, rising inexorably to meet our full potential, and that this collective hero's journey is the "supreme end of man's endeavour."

Near the end of the podcast episode discussing BPD, another therapist, Deborah Stewart, observed how those diagnosed with it can suffer greatly, and that treating clinicians need to draw on equally great reserves of compassion to aid their patients' recovery. "I find myself really moved by this," Stewart then said, "realising the humanity and the telos of where this could be going – into a capacity for relatedness, a capacity for empathy and intuitive sensitivity."

It reminds me of something Eliza had said when I asked what she needed in order to stay well. "I have a community and a support network. Which is why peer work is so important – having people that haven't been through what you've been through but they've experienced similar things or understand what some of it could be like and have empathy." She was silent for a long moment. "Finding your community, your people, having that sense of belonging, which I hadn't felt before. I hadn't felt like I had a culture, or people, or place."

*

Berry Street's CEO, Michael Perusco, has an earnest, almost boyish, face. But because of the nature and extent of his experience with homelessness (he was previously CEO of the St Vincent de Paul Society in New South Wales and the Sacred Heart Mission), I assume there's nothing about the mental health system that could shock him. I am wrong.

During his first week in the role at Berry Street, a young person they were caring for was raped in the community. "I remember thinking, 'Okay, there's going to be a team dedicated to ensuring that support is provided in order to address not just … that immediate trauma, but the ongoing impact,'" he says, explaining that although he wasn't that naive, this was still his first thought. "What was clear was that there was no way that was happening. The current resources that are available, that's the support this young person gets. And that was largely from people who were very well-meaning but not trained in the way to deal with that really complex issue."

Perusco came to Berry Street through his interest in chronic homelessness. Over his career, he had seen that, regardless of age, if someone was experiencing chronic homelessness, they had also experienced childhood trauma. Childhood trauma wasn't simply correlated with chronic homelessness; it was a key driver of it. He wanted the opportunity to work in earlier intervention. "And I guess," he says, "three years into the role, my only conclusion is that I can see exactly why this system delivers that outcome."

Perusco says that there is not yet an effective recognition that children are primary, not secondary, victims of family violence. "It's assumed that they'll just kind of make their way in school and in the world. There isn't much support available for them. So we really can't be that surprised that you're going to have that cohort who are chronically, deeply entrenched in disadvantage. And it manifests itself in homelessness, in mental health, in drugs and alcohol, in crime, in hospitalisation, in the use of ambulances, police, in so many different ways. And what happens in the service system is we all try and deal with it from our own particular lenses, rather than taking a holistic approach and saying, 'What is the need of this person?'"

Children who witness family violence in the household are more likely to re-engage with the justice system in the future, either as a victim or a perpetrator. Seventy-seven per cent of children who witnessed a police-reported family violence incident in 2013–14 went on to have another interaction with the justice system within five years. In 2018–19, one in fifty Victorian children witnessed a family violence incident that was attended by police. Despite the implementation of the Royal Commission into Family Violence's recommendation to prioritise funding for children's counselling, Liana Buchanan, Victoria's principal commissioner for children and young people, has stated that there is still a "serious lack" of therapeutic support for children who have experienced family violence.

So too for sexual violence, as a case that's come up this week – a girl under ten who has been sexually assaulted – demonstrates. "She's come into care, and the response has been to get a roof over her head and work to support carers to manage the placement. But it's not like there's a team of people working intensively to provide a very young girl with the support to recover from what is horrific sexual abuse. What the system delivers is a placement, whether it's in foster care, kinship care or residential care. And things are left to largely work themselves out." He urges me to consider the situation as though it was an adult who had been raped. "Think about the support needs that adult would have. It can be a life-destroying experience. What we're talking about is the case where it's young kids. I think there's an assumption that that care is provided. Everyone's trying to do the best they can within the resources that they've got, but three weeks after coming into care, she hasn't seen her sexual assault therapist."

Between 2019 and 2020, sixty-five children in Victoria who were known to child protection authorities died; five of the deaths were the result of assault, twenty-seven were suicides. The Productivity Commission heard that, in Victoria, only 20 per cent of children who stayed in the child protection system for at least three months between 2010 and 2015 had any type of mental health consultation. There is a National Framework, which includes standards for out-of-home care, yet no national data on adherence to those standards – an eloquent absence.

"When the state removes a child from their family," Perusco explains, "that is one of the most significant decisions our governments make on our behalf. And we can't lose sight of that as a community. We delegate that responsibility to our governments and we assume, for the most part, that it's done well. The reality is that it's not.

"Convincing the people who hold the purse strings in government to invest significantly in this group of people is really tough. There aren't the votes in it."

*

A few months later, Eliza stops on the footpath to google the quickest way to the good café. As we walk down Richmond's narrow back streets on this morning, it occurs to me that I am old enough to be her mother. We pass the Melbourne Clinic – the country's largest private mental health service – and I suddenly think back to when I was her age.

At that time, the medication I had been prescribed by a psychiatrist for severe anxiety and depression made the light hurt my eyes. This medication made my hands tremble so badly that I could not hold a pen. I was ashamed of this tremor. Though I was unable to leave the house much of the time, I was ashamed to ask for special consideration at university. And then I was ashamed of the marks on my transcript, which, if plotted on a graph, would look like a cardiogram. For a decade, I had far more bad days than good; my distress and loneliness were enormous. I thought I would never be able to keep a job or engage with the world I had previously been so eager to embrace. And I thought that would be my life.

Only when I found a therapist who placed my symptoms in their historical context did they begin to subside. This is how I learnt the language of family systems and relational trauma. They gave me an emotional vocabulary and the support I needed to give myself permission to use it. Without my ability to afford continuing sessions – an ability that comes down to privilege and luck – I would probably have been unable to write this essay. I have publicly discussed this previously, and still telling you is difficult. I fear the discrediting stigma which attaches to mental illness in this country. But, as Jung said, nobody is immune to a nationwide evil unless he is unshakably convinced of the danger to his own character of being tainted by the same evil. So I have chosen my fear of that stigma over silence in the face of it. Which is all to say that as Eliza and I walk into the good café and order our coffees, as we discuss deep work and self-compassion, I am listening to her on two levels. The first is with the interest of the 42-year-old author of this essay, watching how Eliza embodies decades of evidence that the negative outcomes associated with BPD might be mediated, or even reversed, with favourable environmental influences such as reparative relationships and cognitive processing of one's experiences. The second is with the admiration of the distressed eighteen-year-old who hadn't attained the insights Eliza has and was convinced, because of those who saw symptoms, not causes, that she never would.

"There's a quote I say all the time," Eliza says, sliding her cup neatly into its saucer. "You can't heal in the environment that made you sick."

THE PUNISHMENT OF DAYLIA MAY BROWN

When eighteen-year-old Daylia May Brown lit a fire among a display of picnic rugs in Target shortly before Christmas in 2018, the law treated BPD as different to any other mental illness or disorder. Brown was an extremely ill teenager who loved art. *The Australian* would later reduce her to insectile proportions in reporting on the Victorian Court of Appeal's "stunning decision" to free "a firebug."

*

"By definition, of course, we believe the person with a stigma is not quite human," wrote Erving Goffman. "On this assumption we exercise varieties of discrimination, through which we effectively, if often unthinkingly, reduce his life chances."

It was Susan Sontag who observed how the "charge of stigmatization" moved from cancer to AIDS, noting that "it seems that societies need to have one illness which becomes identified with evil, and attached blame to its 'victims,' but it is hard to be obsessed with more than one." Here is how we remembered it for our criminal law exams at Melbourne Law School in the late 1990s: *bad not mad*. It referred to the fact that BPD, uniquely, did not count for the purposes of exoneration or mitigation. A little pitchfork of a rhyme.

*

BPD is estimated to affect between 1 and 4 per cent of Australians. Women are three times more likely to be diagnosed with it (or to seek treatment) than men. The name is vestigial, a signifier of early taxonomic uncertainty (whether it was a neurosis or psychosis). Mystery persists in current aetiological conflicts about the independent and interactive roles of biology and environment. A psychiatrist who specialises in the personality disorders tells me the research supports a strong genetic basis. A psychologist who also specialises in personality disorders tells me it is always related to early childhood trauma. The two are not necessarily at odds if it is true that the seeds of emotional and social impairment fall on fertile soil. There are neurobiological hypotheses that emotional regulation is both an individual and an interpersonal process, and that relationships play an important role in regulating biology and behaviour across the lifespan.

Personality disorders are generated in the first years of life, the experienced psychologist explains to me. The different types of personality disorder are connected to the level of cognitive development over that period, but none of the experiences are remembered through the language system, which only develops later. They are instead remembered "in the body." "This means that the baby and the adult into which it develops can have strong emotional responses to events without knowing what has triggered them."

Early disturbances can damage the developing Self, so that there is no clear locus of responsibility for anti-social behaviour (no development in the frontal brain of full "executive function"). "The mind's main means of response to painful stimuli at that stage is dissociation or, if wider structures are involved, splitting," the psychologist continues. "In either case the Self, as it develops later, does not accept a system of responses which seems like a foreign intrusion or which, in other cases, is unconsciously dreaded but not known, let alone understood. It follows that those foreign responses can have a powerful effect on behaviour without the growing and knowing Self taking responsibility for them." The person knows that it is he or she who feels something or does something, but those responses have no connection to the person they consider themself to be, so they don't feel directly responsible. They may attempt to control or limit these "foreign responses," notably with drugs or alcohol, which only compounds their distress. "He or she is struggling with a problem which has no handles.

"Some early intrusions can inhibit the child's ability to see other people as having minds and the intentions they contain," the psychologist says, about the way in which BPD can impact empathy. "There are clinicians who regard this as the defining feature of borderline disorder." This can easily lead to personality disorders being confused with autism or other spectrum disorders.

Childhood abuse and neglect are associated with a range of psycho-pathological outcomes, and neurobiologists continue to investigate why some vulnerable children exposed to risk develop BPD while others don't. There is also evidence of non-traumatic pathways to BPD. What can be said, however, is that those with the diagnosis are neither bad nor mad: they are instead significantly impaired. And there can be a direct causal link between that impairment and criminal behaviour. It's a complex area, and the history of medical uncertainty did the law no favours.

*

Three years before Brown walked through the city with her matches, legal academic Jamie Walvisch was reading a Victorian appeal court judgment with the definite feeling that something was wrong. It was the 2015 case of Michael O'Neill, forty-eight, who had received eighteen years' imprisonment with a non-parole period of thirteen years for murdering his partner, Stuart Rattle. Following an argument early one Wednesday morning, O'Neill strangled Rattle with a dog lead and placed his body in a furniture bag on their bed. Then he showered and went to work in their downstairs office, maintaining – over the next five days – a pretence that Rattle was alive. On Sunday evening, he ordered takeaway, set out dinner for two and placed a lit candle too close to the curtains near the body on the bed. Then he went to buy something sweet, returning to see his apartment on fire. Not ablaze enough, however, to destroy the evidence.

In the psychological report he was diagnosed with dependant personality disorder with prominent features of narcissistic personality disorder. He was sentenced in the Supreme Court, where Justice Elizabeth Hollingsworth recounted some of his history, saying that his relationship with Rattle was complex and needed to be understood against the background of his childhood and psychological make-up. "You are someone who was cut off emotionally from an incredibly young age, who never came to terms with your sexuality, and who was bullied as a child because of it. The coping mechanisms which you learnt as a child were avoidance, detachment, and (ultimately) dependence." Born in Ireland, he was the second-youngest of five children. The family moved to Australia when he was five, settling in country Victoria. His father was a farmer. Much of his mother's time was spent caring for an intellectually disabled sibling, without family support.

> You were frequently teased and bullied, both at home and at school, for being "girly" or "a poof." Sometimes the bullying was physical, as well as verbal. Even though you identified yourself at an early age as being exclusively homosexual, you had great trouble coming to terms with that fact ... In the 16 years that you were in a relationship with Mr Rattle, you never once introduced him to your family ... Mr Rattle ... had a dominant, controlling personality; everything had to be done his way, both personally and professionally ... In front of others, he would call you lazy, a parasite; he would threaten to send you back to where you came from ...

To be not guilty of a crime by reason of mental impairment, the defence must prove that the person was so ill he did not know the wrongfulness of his actions. It's an extremely high threshold and was irrelevant to O'Neill's case, as he pleaded guilty. Mental impairment can, however, also be taken into consideration to mitigate a sentence. The principles governing that process derive from a case called *Verdins*. The Verdins principles state that a mental disorder, abnormality or impairment may influence a sentence in various ways. It may reduce moral culpability (as distinct from legal responsibility). It may influence the type of sentence imposed and the conditions in which it is served. It may moderate or eliminate the need to impose a sentence intended to deter similar behaviour in others, a mentally unwell offender not being an appropriate "vehicle" (in the bloodless language of the law) for that message. Similarly, it may moderate or eliminate the need to impose a sentence intended to deter that particular offender from reoffending, given the effect of his condition on his judgment. Last, it may call for a reduction in the severity of the sentence, given that the conditions under which it would be served would weigh more heavily on the offender than on a person with better health.

Given the frequency of mental illness among those who come into contact with our criminal justice system, it is unsurprising that *Verdins* is the most cited appellate case in Victoria. Defence lawyers have raised its principles in relation to everything from depression caused by the offender's own offending to the effects of chronic physical pain. However, BPD was uniquely excluded from the expansive ambit of those principles. Whether it was describing brain chemicals, or genetics, or the sequelae of complex trauma, the moralising language of agency and choice was employed for discussing personality disorder.

In Victoria, the starkest example of this long-held position is the case of Garry David in the late 1980s and early '90s. From the activity of their eyebrows and the silent O shaped by their lips, it seems that the ghost of Garry David haunts the collective consciousness of Victorians over a certain age, all of whom remember how "crazy" he was, how dangerous, but few of whom know just how brutal his childhood was, before and after he was removed from home at the age of four to be raised largely by the state. Following the medical understanding at the time, the personality disorders with which David had been diagnosed were excluded from the legislative definitions of "mental illness." Therefore, despite the egregious harm he continued to inflict on himself and which he envisaged inflicting on "a community that would not help him to become part of it," he could not be detained for medical treatment. Nor could he be detained for punishment, having served his time for previous offending. So the government passed ad hominem legislation to enable only Garry David to be detained for the protection of the community.

Against this jurisprudential history, when Hollingworth found that O'Neill's personality disorder had "played some role" in his offending, and therefore operated to mitigate his moral culpability and, to a certain extent, his suitability as a vehicle for deterring others – the Director of Public Prosecutions predictably took issue. In the ensuing appeal, the state successfully argued that the Verdins principles didn't apply because O'Neill's "personality disorder did not affect his capacity to reason, or to rationally make decisions." Bad not mad.

"It seemed based on a completely flawed understanding of the nature of personality disorders, and how impairing they can be," Walvish, whose specialisation is sentencing, says about his reaction to the appeal decision. Given the current medical understanding of personality disorders, there was no principled reason to distinguish them from other mental disorders, he explains. "Part of the sentencing process should be about tailoring the sentence to the particular needs of the offender. To say that personality disorders aren't really relevant means that you're going to be precluded from appropriately tailoring a sentence in that way. So not just from a question of principle but also from a practical perspective, it was going to have consequences for a very large number of people." While the data is still unclear, it appears that the proportion of offenders with personality disorders could be around 40 per cent.

The lack of a more nuanced approach threw into question the basis for conclusions regarding blameworthiness, impacts of imprisonment, risk of reoffending and the likely effectiveness of rehabilitative interventions. In addition to the history of medical uncertainty in the area, Walvish explains that underlying factors were at play. "I think what happened after *Verdins* was there was this explosion of cases where mental health problems were suddenly raised in almost every sentencing case before the courts. Very often on the basis of quite poor-quality evidence. So, in the background you had this sense of judicial disquiet that things had gotten a little bit out of control."

With forensic psychiatrist Andrew Carroll, Walvish began to raise awareness about the need to change the law to reflect contemporary scientific understandings of personality pathologies. Approaching Victoria Legal Aid, they met with Tim Marsh, then Chief Counsel, to discuss pushing the matter in the courts. That requires a sympathetic litigant. Marsh put out a call to Legal Aid lawyers, but it would be another year before a solicitor – looking at the arson charges against a teenager who had offended because she felt safer in prison – would say, "I think we found her."

In the absence of legislative action, change was going to have to come from the appeal court recognising that its previous decision – a recent one – was wrong. And because of skilful use of expert information, that's exactly what happened. At bottom, however, change happens when the legal system recognises that without necessary self-correction it will lose public confidence in the administration of justice.

At this point, I should tell you that extending Verdins to people with BPD is "a wind that blows both ways," to use a phrase of Marsh's. The argument that an offender is so unwell that they cannot be held fully morally responsible for their actions means the court may mitigate punishment on those grounds. However, by making that argument, counsel risk effectively conceding that their client's dysregulation makes them a public safety risk, and consequently punishment can be increased on the grounds of dangerousness.

*

Sitting in the Magistrates' Court in June 2019, I saw 21-year-old Codey Herrmann's face pop up via video link and immediately thought that he looked simultaneously very young and very old. During the short hearing – during which he pleaded guilty to the rape and murder of 21-year-old Aiia Maasarwe, involving violence so catastrophic before he burnt her body that her family successfully moved for the details to be suppressed to preserve her dignity – he was jarringly cooperative. With a gesture that's become more familiar if not less awkward, he gave the magistrate a tiny wave before the screen went blank. Herrmann was diagnosed with a severe personality disorder. In October 2019, he was sentenced by

Justice Hollingworth. Marsh, Herrmann's counsel, stated that he had no prior convictions, no history of violence, that there was no simple explanation for his actions, but that it was necessary to consider his background to understand how he came to be the damaged young man who committed his offences.

"Much of your life history has been extensively documented in more than 2000 pages of welfare records, in your file kept by the Victorian Aboriginal Child Care Agency," Hollingworth stated, in her judgment.

> There is no doubt that the environment in which you lived for the first three years of your life was one of extreme physical and emotional deprivation. By the time you were six months old, you had come to the attention of welfare authorities, due to your mother's alcohol problems and maternal violence. You were temporarily removed from your parents. By your first birthday, your mother had abandoned you into the care of a relative whose own children had been removed by court order due to serious neglect. About six months later, you were again taken into care, and hospitalised with scabies. Over the next eighteen months, while living with one or both of your parents, you were the subject of numerous welfare notifications, due to chronic parental drug and alcohol problems, domestic violence, emotional abuse, and failure to meet your basic needs (including adequate food). The level of physical neglect was so profound that you and your sister had digestive problems, rotten teeth, and skin problems due to lack of cleanliness. You also had delayed developmental milestones . . .
>
> After beginning school in 2004, you soon displayed a range of behavioural problems. You were emotionally fragile, with anger and self-esteem issues. You had difficulty forming friendships and negotiating social play situations. You were often rough or aggressive with other children, and had difficulty controlling your behaviour. You also had poor concentration in class. Your mother died when you were 13. That coincided with a steady decline in

your behaviour. Anger, cannabis and alcohol abuse, and truanting from school, began to emerge as problems … By late 2014, you had begun leaving your foster home and sleeping rough … Your first recorded involvement with mental health services was in November 2016, when you were admitted as an inpatient to Orygen Youth Health, because you were floridly psychotic.

Herrmann continued to decline; he was living in transitional youth housing and dropped out of school in Year 11. In June 2018, he tried to return to his foster mother, but was unable to stop using drugs, so he moved out in September, becoming homeless. "You have only ever had brief periods of casual employment in unskilled jobs," Hollingworth continued. "Your social contacts were limited to a small group of people, all of whom were also abusing substances. You were not particularly close to anybody … About one month before this offending, you had attempted suicide …"

Marsh argued that the Verdins principles did in fact apply to Herrmann. Hollingworth agreed. And then that wind blew both ways through the court: Herrmann's moral culpability was reduced because of his background of deprivation and his mental disorder, while the need to protect the public from him was heightened. He received thirty-six years' imprisonment, a duration longer than the time he has been alive. That sentence was too high for some people, given his childhood experiences, too low for others, given his monstrous offending. But you cannot read about the factors that formed him without seeing the uncomfortable truth that monsters are always human.

"We don't focus about the revenge," Aiia Maasarwe's father, Saeed, said outside court. "This is not our compass, this is not our focus, but to care for the society, for the people, for the ladies [to be able to] go out and go back home."

*

I learnt about First Steps from Tania Wolff, the president of the Law Institute of Victoria and a sessional member of the Mental Health Tribunal, who works there. It's a one-stop shop providing medical care and legal advice, and its clients are predominantly people with profound affect dysregulation due to a mix of trauma, mental illness and addiction. Established in 2008, it did not receive government funding until 2020.

Wolff, a self-described optimist, is heartened by the increased recognition that vulnerable groups are overrepresented in the criminal justice system and that prison does very little to reduce offending. But, she says, as a community we have a lot of work to do in changing our view of those who break the law. Here, she brings up an example that causes me to think of Herrmann.

"Years ago there was that horrendous atrocity, in Oslo," she says, referring to the seventy-seven people murdered by Anders Breivik in 2011. "It was the biggest trauma that country had ever experienced, that huge massacre of children. The equivalent of the chief commissioner of their police went in front of the national media and said something we would never hear. That was, effectively: we, as a society, have a part in this as well; we have a responsibility for this because there were multiple moments where there was a potential intervention in this person's life ... and we'd missed all of those moments."

Wolff is influenced by the Hungarian-Canadian physician Gabor Maté, who set up the equivalent of First Steps in Vancouver. Underlying most of the mental health and addiction issues that her clients have, she explains, is trauma and pain. "Maté said that when we talk about addiction, we ask the wrong question. We ask, 'Why the addiction?' but we need to be asking instead, 'Why the pain?' He talks about the fact that alcohol was the first analgesic. Heroin, all of the opiates are painkillers. His patients – and my clients – those who are in this cycle of addiction, are searching for escape from pain. What we as a community have to do is work out better ways of creating opportunities and space for people to be healed."

*

The quietly radical step – of considering the impact of Herrmann's mental disorder on his blameworthiness – that had already been taken in his sentencing (and would be confirmed in a subsequent appeal) was elevated to the level of principle through the accident of timing and the choice of "vehicle." Given the extreme violence of Herrmann's offending, he was not a sympathetic litigant – fair enough, though the phrase says more about those doing the emoting than those receiving it. It happened that Daylia May Brown – whose case was listed shortly after Herrmann's – was young like he was, and diagnosed with a personality disorder like he was. Unlike Herrmann, she had a criminal history and no evidence of a background of extreme deprivation. However, her offending didn't involve direct interpersonal violence and she was female. Plus, it strikes me, though no one I interviewed mentioned it, she was white.

*

A joyless Alice moved through a dark Wonderland behind the glass of the Myer windows, and Christmas music jangled in the shops as Brown walked through the city on the evening of 18 December 2018. She had recently turned eighteen, adulthood arriving suddenly with all its baggage at her door. *I'll be home for Christmas* . . . Based on what the court would later hear, it appears that the youth prison where Brown had been sent at sixteen – after burning down her hometown's only supermarket – occupied the emotional terrain usually associated with home. She had recently been released from that prison into supported accommodation, from which she'd absconded. During her two weeks of freedom, she'd used $1000 worth of methamphetamine. Experienced hallucinations, believed people were trying to kill her, carried a blade to defend herself. She'd thought, a few times, about setting fires. The matches and aerosol deodorant she held as she stood in the Target shop on Bourke Street were her ticket back to what had become familiar. She lit the picnic rugs first, then a display of cosmetic bags. The first fire was quickly extinguished by staff, only for them to realise that the second fire had been lit. The store was evacuated and the fire brigade extinguished the flames.

Meanwhile, Brown had walked to a Coles supermarket, where she threw a lit match into the shelves of female sanitary products and left. She returned a short time later, watched the flames, left again. She went to a Woolworths nearby, took some toilet roll from a shelf, lit it in the aisle with baby products and walked away. Shortly after, staff noticed the burnt-out toilet roll, which had not done serious damage.

Thin, young, long dark hair. She was easily identified from CCTV footage and found outside Flinders Street Station by two protective services officers. After being forced to the ground and handcuffed, Brown kicked out at one of the officers, striking them in the shin. She would be charged with resisting arrest and assaulting an emergency worker. Due to her mental state, she was unable to be interviewed by police. So she was taken to the Royal Melbourne Hospital emergency department and then transferred to Orygen, where she was admitted to the psychiatric unit.

On 22 December, Brown called the police and told them she was going to burn down the Queen Victoria Building because she wanted to go to jail. "I don't deserve to be in this world," she told the psychiatrist, "I need to be punished. There is no hope for me in this world. Everyone has given up on me. I do want to change and be better, but I don't think that can happen." After slashing her leg with glass and trying to cut her wrist, she was secluded and restrained, with olanzapine in her muscles, screaming that she wanted police to be called, that she wanted to go to prison.

A few days later, she was discharged to supported accommodation in Brunswick under the full-time supervision of a mental health organisation. However, she was driven to the police station that same day by a case worker after repeating threats to burn down the QV building. She was again detained by police, again taken to the Royal Melbourne Hospital emergency department, again released back to supported accommodation. Notes from a medical review around this time stated that part of the motivation for fire-setting had been to return to youth custody, but that wasn't the whole picture; "It sometimes felt satisfying, as though I've completed something, that's how it's meant to end, to play out, that's just life ..."

Around 2 am on Saturday, 29 December, Brown broke a window to enter an empty house in Travancore, where she had previously lived. The house was owned by the Department of Justice and Community Safety and used as an outpatient mental health facility. Once inside, she stacked a chair on a table and climbed up, reaching towards the ceiling to light the insulation in the roof. She then lit some bedding and left. From the dark of a nearby school, she watched the house go up in flames. She was seen nearby around 2:30 am and arrested. She told the police what she had done and was taken to the Melbourne Custody Centre. At processing, she reported that there was a razorblade in her bra, and denied concealing anything else. However, after a further instruction to remove any concealed razors, she handed over another razorblade. This would result in another charge of taking a weapon into a prison. She was still on remand in adult prison fifteen months later due to the government's inability to find suitable housing.

"Her life has been blighted," said Judge Mark Taft in the Victorian County Court when sentencing Brown in March 2020. "She was affected by reasonably severe anorexia nervosa in early adolescence and since then has suffered from extremely fragile self-esteem and complex personality deficits. Ms Brown has an extensive history of self-harm and multiple hospital admissions. During the course of this proceeding, Ms Brown has been hospitalised as a result of cutting herself with sharp blades and swallowing a spoon whilst in custody."

The week before, Brown appeared in court straight after being released from the Alfred Hospital. She would tell Marsh, her lawyer, "I feel like I don't have a place in the world, I just want to disappear and die."

Psychiatrist Andrew Carroll had prepared for the court an enormously comprehensive report detailing Brown's history, explaining his diagnosis of "severe personality disorder with detachment and a borderline pattern," and elaborating on his opinion that her offending directly related to that mental disorder. As a document, Marsh would explain to me later, it spoke eloquently to Brown's issues while also functioning as a masterclass in the evolution of the medical understanding of personality disorders for its true and future audience, the Court of Appeal.

Taft emphasised that Brown's sentencing was delayed because, despite funding being in place, the government's inability to provide her with housing caused the proceedings to be adjourned. And adjourned again. And again and again and again. This delay, Taft stated, "exacerbated Ms Brown's anxiety and has increased her risk of self-harm." Describing her personal circumstances, Taft noted that Brown's mother had supported her in court and that contact with her father was sporadic. Her parents separated when she was around seven. Taft mentioned that "there appears to have been considerable interpersonal conflict between her parents during her childhood." No evidence was provided of a history of abuse or neglect.

Brown's mother noticed a change in her daughter around eight years old. She became shyer and started struggling at school. She would answer questions with single-word answers, usually pertaining to a rodent or other animal. Her mother was told about an incident when her daughter alleged that she was held down and touched inappropriately by some boys, but was unable to find out more. One clinician the family consulted appeared to assume that Brown was a survivor of childhood sexual abuse, but there was no evidence to support that belief. She began self-harming in high school. She also suffered from an eating disorder and had regular contact with mental health services. Taft stated that Brown "effectively disengaged from schooling in Year 7." Her Year 8 coordinator described her as the "guru for the disaffected kids," and said that she seemed like Gollum from The Lord of the Rings, wanting contact with others but then being afraid of them. Brown dropped out of school in Year 8.

One summer night in 2016, when she was fifteen, after several weeks of feeling weird and angry, Brown burnt down the IGA in Beechworth, orange flames roiling behind the wall of broken windows out front. This was the first fire that she set, she told Carroll. There had been an altercation with the family of a boy she had been friendly with and she subsequently developed homicidal thoughts regarding another boy who, some years earlier, had "got into her space" at school. After telling her therapist that she was having homicidal and suicidal thoughts, she was admitted to the adolescent unit at Box Hill Hospital. It was there that she started thinking about fire. She was discharged three days before the incident. She said that she settled on the supermarket because "it was the biggest in the town, the food source for everyone. I wanted to burn the whole town."

Brown was found not guilty on the grounds of mental impairment for the charges related to the IGA fire. However, instead of being treated in a therapeutic setting, she was detained in youth prison – the Melbourne Youth Justice Centre in Parkville – because the magistrate at the Wodonga Children's Court was satisfied that there was no practicable alternative. In October 2018, Brown was admitted to the high dependency unit at the Royal Children's Hospital and absconded by climbing over a fence.

The list, in Carroll's report, of Brown's episodes of self-harm and hospital admissions from the age of fourteen is long, distressing and deeply sad. There were at least three suicide attempts. Discussing the factors underlying the conduct for which she was arrested, Carroll emphasised that Brown longed for a return to Parkville, that the prison had become a place she was emotionally attached to. That it was probably not a coincidence that the city fires occurred a fortnight after she turned eighteen, Brown progressively having learnt that, for her, fire setting was associated with a gratifying sense of being able to exert control over a world she found "frightening, threatening and alien as a result of her personality dysfunction."

Taft devoted a great deal of space in his judgment to setting out the professional opinions of both Carroll and Professor James Ogloff, executive director of psychological services and research at the Victorian Institute of Forensic Mental Health, that the legal position on BPD was incorrect, based on outdated clinical understandings and required reconsideration as a matter of accuracy and fairness. It was Carroll's clinical opinion that Brown's personality disorder had a "very significant" impact on her ability to exercise appropriate judgment. It also prevented her from experiencing the inhibitory mechanisms that others would, and from having an emotional awareness that the conduct was wrong on a "deeper moral level." While imprisonment initially had a positive impact in removing her from risk factors in the community, Carroll described continued incarceration as counterproductive for her rehabilitation and risk mitigation in the long term. Brown would eventually suffer more than the average prisoner because of her personality disorder. He pointed to her attempts to return to custody as an early manifestation of institutionalisation. If he was describing any other diagnosis, all of this would have provided impetus for strong mitigation. But it was not any other diagnosis.

Finding that the legal orthodoxy regarding BPD effectively tied his hands, Taft reluctantly imposed a prison sentence of eighteen months. But he did not go gently. He stated that were it not for those restrictions, Verdins principles would have "materially reduced" Brown's sentence. He spoke directly to Brown, which, in itself, is not rare; the judicial role is intended to personify the power of the state. But his tone, the register he used, felt extraordinary. "Can I speak to you briefly, Daylia," Taft said. "You need not stand. I rather doubt that there is anything I can say that will make you happier about your connection with the world or allow you to feel better about yourself. I wish I could. All I can do is give you an end date for your imprisonment and hope that the housing and supports that are in place will assist you in the future ..." I believe there was a moral drive for his direct address to Brown. But Taft's main audience was the appeal court, to whom he would deliver immediate notice of his decision so that they could speedily overturn him – and themselves.

*

Like judges, barristers are cloaked and rarefied creatures. Their hair is as vulnerable to disappointments as ours, but it is frequently hidden under their wigs, which range from snow white to tobacco-smoked yellow. Their clothes get wrinkled too but are often concealed under the dark materials of their robes. And the fact that their offices (commercially carpeted, white MDF walled, same as any suburban accountant) go by the audaciously rococo name "chambers" obscures the mundane grind of much of their daily work and the lineball calls – moral, legal and strategic – that attend it as they grapple with laws written by fallible humans.

Tim Marsh, the barrister who represented Brown and Herrmann, has a strong interest in mental impairment and disability law. He has represented some of the nation's most notorious offenders (Gerald Ridsdale, Jaymes Todd) and has received death threats for that work. In addition to his law degree, Marsh completed a science degree, majoring in genetics. Before legal practice, he spent nearly a decade working as a software developer. This interest in concealed coding is reflected in the submissions he drafts regarding his clients' mental, moral and medical states, and by the human anatomical posters hanging near the desk behind which he is sitting, answering the question I've just asked by challenging the assumption on which it is based. My question concerned the biographical details he'd provided to the court in his sentencing plea on Brown's behalf. Compared with verbal portraits he'd painted of Herrmann and others for this purpose, it seemed conspicuously lacking in evidence of childhood deprivation or trauma that could explain the anti-social behaviour of the young woman with the scar of a self-inflicted wound across her throat.

"I think there are some interesting points of comparison between her and Codey Herrmann," Marsh says, "in the sense that in Codey's case you had this quite breathtaking neglect from the ages of zero to three that you could very much hang your hat on in terms of saying that's the aetiology of the personality disorder. In Daylia's case, it was simply less clear what the origin was. It might not have been the most socially advantaged upbringing, but it wasn't abusive or neglectful. So it was something of a mystery why she ended up as profoundly socially excluded as she was, and as profoundly impaired." This conforms with what Andrew Chanen, at Orygen, had told me: while trauma is very common among people with BPD, it is neither necessary nor sufficient to develop the disorder.

"When we see somebody as vulnerable as Daylia engaging in such profound acts of self-harm, sabotaging her life in order to go to custody, we want to know [if] that's in response to something terrible that's happened," Marsh continues. "And what if it's not? What if that's just how some of us turn out? How does that make us feel?

"I think your question is entirely reasonable," he says. "It hints at the human desire for all of this stuff to make sense. We all want to feel safe. We want to have an explanation."

The data on juries – our collective representatives – demonstrates that the more information they have, the less punitive they are. That's generally true of you and me and everyone else, including judges, which is why the marshalling and communication of humanising context is one of Marsh's highest duties. Yet one of the things that makes him so interesting as an advocate is that he doesn't shy away from the white space in the narratives he constructs. We don't have a high tolerance for the discomfort of these unknowns. If the stories we tell ourselves about the world can be compared to houses, unknowns are the basements and attics and sheds we fill with the detritus collected over a lifetime: fear and blame and rage. By clearing that space, Marsh's candour works counterintuitively to elicit grace. I have seen him do this in court. There is a change of atmosphere when he touches on what can only be described as the human mystery. And while it remains true that when it comes to environmental causal factors, absence of evidence is not evidence of absence, it is also true that the effect of Marsh's manner is an unlikely collective softening into sorrow.

Because Marsh deals daily with tragedy, he is ideally placed to discern patterns and pathologies in our institutions. "I'm seeing people who've committed serious criminal offences, who are statistically a fairly small proportion of people living with a mental illness," he says. "Having said that, if I had to narrate the platonic ideal of clients I get, I can tell you that they will have family who have struggled to get them into treatment. There will be a history of lack of follow-up and service disengagement. Chronic instability of housing, undeniable warning signs in an escalation of seriousness, but an inability of services to properly respond." He sees "the ongoing human toll for lack of intervention at a point in time where it could have made a difference."

"We have a justice system that's more or less optimised for apportioning individual responsibility," he says. Think of ripples radiating outwards on a pond. "At the very centre, you have individual responsibility, and you can apportion that pretty readily. Then the next ring out, you have institutional responsibility. What are the institutions that could have, or should have, supported this person? Then the outermost ring is societal, or collective responsibility." He says that if the criminal justice system engages with the concept of societal responsibility, he can't see it.

"So what's the question with Jaymes Todd and Codey Herrmann that's unanswered in all of this? I think that question is: how does a nineteen-year-old with no priors fall through? How does a nineteen-year-old get to a point of acknowledging that their life is so bleak and so meaningless that, at that age, they have already passed their apogee of existence and it's downhill from here? That they know, deep down, that it's never going to be better and they literally have nothing to risk? So the question that's not being asked is: what's the value of the social contract when it's only operating in one way?

"It's convenient to want to demonise the individual but I think a much bigger question is to ask: what happens when there are people who have nothing to lose? What level of risk can we embrace? Can we tolerate having people in our midst who have no possibility of a meaningful future? It's just – 'I'm not part of this world.'

"That's something that really weighs heavily on me because I've seen it repeatedly. Codey Herrmann, like Jaymes Todd, destroyed his own life as deliberately as he took somebody else's; he was never getting away with it. Why does someone do that? And why don't we care?" It's not a lack of understanding that's stopping earlier interventions, Marsh continues. "It's the presence of a dual disability. Or 'we can't help you, because they've got an alcohol problem too.' Of course they do. 'Oh, well, this person doesn't have a stable address.' Housing is a foundational issue. Look at every area mental health service – the clue's in the title: 'area.' If you're homeless, or transient, you don't fall within it." There are so many examples where the problems are known, he says, but "the System" operates in such a way as to prevent the taking of responsibility. "Mental health and disability issues aren't like fine wine. They don't get better if you lay them down for a while. They just get worse. And disadvantage compounds.

"The inevitability about this is that we collectively end up paying anyway. We can pay with involuntary treatment and mental health services for the most at-risk people. We can pay by providing purpose-built facilities for people with certain disorders. Or we can pay with suffering, endless incarceration, needless death. We will pay, one way or the other."

*

Appeals are typically heard by three judges. In Brown's case, however, a bench of five was convened. In August 2020, they reversed their earlier categorical exclusion of personality disorders from the Verdins framework. As the court stated in Brown's appeal, quoting from *Verdins*, a diagnostic label should be treated as the beginning, not the end, of the enquiry.

In his evidence, Carroll emphasised that, as regards the severity of impairment or distress, there was no relevant distinction between personality disorder and other mental health conditions. On the contrary, he said: "I think any experienced psychologist or psychiatrist would tell you that among the most distressed and impaired people that they have worked with over the years of their career ... will be the people with serious personality disorder."

In re-sentencing Brown, the court acknowledged that her pervasive, longstanding disorder had "fundamentally impaired her ability to act rationally, regulate her conduct and fully understand the consequences." Her moral culpability – and consequently, her sentence – was significantly reduced. The best outcome for her was a supportive, therapeutic environment in the community. This was also the best outcome for the community in terms of managing her risk of reoffending. "On that basis, we were satisfied that her incarceration should come to an end at the earliest practicable opportunity."

Ten months later, in June 2021, another five-member bench heard the state's appeal against Herrmann's sentence, brought on the grounds that it was inadequately low. They began by describing the unenviable, perhaps impossible, task of sentencing Herrmann: "The judge's responsibility, on behalf of the community, is to provide a dispassionate assessment both of the objective gravity of the offending and of the subjective culpability of the offender, at the same time acknowledging the pain and distress which the offending has caused."

It's an open secret that the sentencing aim of deterrence is largely specious. Regardless of how harshly a court punishes, it will not force dysregulated individuals into a cost–benefit analysis before acting. The legal fiction is poor protection. Nonetheless, while demanding so little of our other institutions – and the governments we empower to oversee them – we continue to mislocate our hopes for safety in the criminal justice system, which cannot resurrect the dead or prospectively redeem the living.

Given the impact of Herrmann's background and his illness on his moral blameworthiness for his crimes, the state's appeal was denied. All going well, Herrmann will be eligible for parole consideration in thirty years, when he is fifty-one.

*

Much of it comes down to this: we do most of our living in old houses. Take the Supreme Court, for example, where Brown and Herrmann's appeals were heard; it was completed in 1884, the year of the Royal Commission on Asylums for the Insane and Inebriate, the public inquiry that made the unheeded recommendation to close the old Yarra Bend Asylum. After being appointed Inspector General of the Insane in 1905, Dr Ernest Jones noted that Yarra Bend's original bluestone building remained in use and that it "must have been designed on the lines of prison galleries." "The airing courts were very small and damnable," he wrote, "with high bluestone walls, preventing all view of the outside country. There was also a row of outside cells, with earth closets, two dark padded cells and an all-pervading smell of poor, mad humanity." It took another twenty years for all the patients to be transferred.

After Yarra Bend was demolished, one of its "ha-ha" walls remained, cut into the earth. Looking up from the inside, this was an insurmountably high wall. From the outside, however, it could barely be discerned on the plane of the earth. The name is thought to have come from the surprise expressed by those discovering the drop that had not been visible until they were nearly over the edge; an invisible divide, a lie of contiguity preserving the preferred image of the landscape. The gateway of the old asylum remained, as did the infirmary which, in 1927, was incorporated into the new Fairhaven Venereal Disease Clinic for women, where "the outcast and diseased," many of them pregnant sex workers, lived. When Fairhaven closed, its wall was incorporated into Fairlea, the women's prison built on the site. In this way, and so many others, the original dark place passed into the next. Fairlea was later razed but some of Yarra Bend's foundations remain underground, as do – most likely – some of its patients' bodily remains in unmarked, common graves near what is currently a pleasant fairway of the Yarra Bend golf course. Now the most visible trace of the state's first mental hospital, where thousands lived and died, is a single gate post.

Directly across a quiet road from that gate post, one grey morning in 2021, Dr Danny Sullivan sits at his desk in Thomas Embling Hospital – Victoria's secure forensic mental health hospital – under a print of Hieronymus Bosch's *Paradise and Hell*. Sullivan is a forensic psychiatrist and the executive director of clinical services at Forensicare, also known as the Victorian Institute of Forensic Mental Health, the provider of mental health services to people living with a serious mental illness in, or at risk of entering, the criminal justice system. Many of his patients are mentally ill people who have committed offences; the diverse cohort of unwell individuals long stigmatised as "the criminally insane."

Sullivan speaks gently and precisely. He is held in high esteem by academics, judges, lawyers and his office mates, it appears, from the joy and frequency with which he is greeted as he leads me from the hospital's reception area to his office, passing through an open-plan workplace which is like any other workplace except that it is situated in a mental hospital. This mundanity may come as a surprise, and that surprise would be instructive for a few reasons. First, it speaks to the fact that the work done by forensic services is, largely, invisible. It takes place in hospitals and prisons, away from the public gaze. To the extent that this work exists in the public imagination, that image is wrong. It is more bureaucratic than gothic. Prison, Sullivan says, is very banal. "It's just people living in a different setting for a significant period of their lives. Going about their usual business, but without the liberty of returning to the community." At this point, we are interrupted by the chirping of a bird, which signals the hour on an Audubon clock hanging high on Sullivan's wall. It is a jarringly familiar sound. I, too, once owned this charming and ridiculous clock and I cannot look at it without feeling the warmth of home. For a moment, we smile up at it with mutual delight.

The second reason the startling ordinariness of forensic mental health is important is that it counters the usual "prurience," Sullivan's word, which surrounds this social milieu. "Those who have committed offences which are spectacular or end up in the media will always attract the fascination of people but [it is] often a fascination teamed with revulsion or anxiety," he says.

The last reason is connected to the first two. "For thousands of years, people with mental illness have been regarded as different," Sullivan says. "Whether it's been possessed by the gods, cursed, afflicted by an illness, afflicted by genetic infirmities, the various narratives have always Othered that population. The confronting thing about mental health discourse these days is the reflection that mental health disorders are incredibly common.

They're distributed throughout the community. They select for people with disadvantage and adverse childhood experiences and marginalisation, but they don't *necessarily* select. There are plenty of people who aren't expecting mental disorder who develop one." That's the problem with prurience, I think, sitting under the bird clock. We squint sneakily through some keyhole expecting to comfort ourselves with the fate of Others, only to find in their dim little rooms the jarringly familiar – just ourselves, waiting.

According to Sullivan, the population at Thomas Embling invariably has a combination of four severe problems: psychotic illness; severe personality problems (many of which are related to a history of deprivation or marginalisation); cognitive impairments (innate or acquired); and substance use disorders. The latter, he explains, "are just so strongly correlated with serious offending that it's undeniable." They are also strongly correlated with deteriorations in mental health and downward trajectories in social adjustment – "accommodation, relationships, access to whatever benefits the society has."

It is this context, Sullivan says, that causes people "to retain a fear and an antipathy towards people with mental disorder … And of course, the antipathy of people towards offending is because they also see it as being committed by Others, despite the fact that we know much violent offending occurs covertly, in domestic relationships. We know that much sexual offending occurs covertly, in domestic relationships. Not from strangers in parks and streets, but rather from family members and trusted adults and invariably against vulnerable children. So I think those narratives affect the way forensic mental health is regarded." Just ourselves, then, waiting.

*

In his study of stigma, Goffman, the sociologist, wrote about its contagiousness. In his classification of relationships to stigma, there are – in addition to the Normals and the Stigmatised – the Wise. Borrowing the term from the mid-century gay community, Goffman explained that the Wise are Normals "whose special situation has made them intimately privy to the secret life of the stigmatized individual and sympathetic with it, and who find themselves accorded a measure of acceptance ... in the clan." The Wise are "the marginal men" before whom the stigmatised need feel no shame, knowing that they will be seen in full and as "an ordinary other." That is, as someone different from, but equal to, the "I" of ourselves – as deserving of respect, and in need of compassion, as we are. In return, the discredit of stigmatisation leaks onto them.

It is noteworthy that it is precisely because Sullivan (like Marsh) is a superbly qualified professional who has not accepted the prepackaged narrative regarding the feared population with whom he works that he is one of Goffman's marginal men. Though much of Sullivan's time is taken up with policy and procedure, working with his patients is the part of his job he enjoys most. "The reason you do medicine, usually, is because you want to work with people," he says. "And the reason you do psychiatry is because you want to work with a particular group of people. The people I most enjoy working with are people with intellectual disability, people with severe psychotic illness and people who have usually engaged in very serious, violent or sexual offending."

When I ask why, he replies, "They're a group of people for whom I feel I've been able to work fairly dispassionately but without being overly influenced by negative thoughts towards them. So I can retain a degree of objectivity." This serves him well with the aspects of his job that require him to provide expert information to courts, tribunals and parole boards. "It means that you can provide opinions which are, hopefully, less tainted by subjective prejudice, and really are focused upon the evidence, the facts and the clinical information which are relevant to legal decisions.

"Of course," he continues, "what people really want is for [these] people to be locked away forever, and never bother them again. And that's not a luxury we have. Our luxury is very much that we have the opportunity to treat people effectively, but the intention is to return them to the community, safely. Some people will not return to the community – they will never be in a situation where they're safe. But it's a fantasy to think that because you are mentally disordered and have committed an offence, that you should therefore be locked away forever."

Because imprisonment has criminogenic effects, those who return to the community from being therapeutically treated at Thomas Embling Hospital have lower recidivism rates than those who are jailed. One of the most striking differences between forensic and public mental healthcare is that, with the former, psychiatrists and patients get the benefit of sustained contact. "Unlike the rapid churn of underfunded public mental health services, where people aren't retained in services or in inpatient units for long enough to develop a relationship with them for them to get better and to sustain their recovery, we get the long story," Sullivan explains. This enables clinicians to truly communicate with these patients. "One of the things most of our patients tell us when they've recovered is that they recognise that they've transgressed in a way they can't ever forget and the community can't forget. If they apply for a job, if they apply for a rental, the stigma of their past will haunt them. So it's really important for us to work constructively with that group – not about how to conceal what's happened, but how do we integrate it into their future life to ensure that they can live safely and return to the community, and live a good life."

I've seen it numerous times now, but I was shocked when I first read in a sentencing judgment that the judge's preferred therapeutic sentence could not be imposed due to a lack of beds. Following the Royal Commission, Thomas Embling's bed numbers have doubled. So while, as Sullivan observes, that increase represents only the normal accretion that should have happened over the past twenty years, it is a sign of some positive change. Another positive change that he's witnessed over the course of his career is an increasing recognition of different narratives by the justice system. "Specifically, the devastating effect of incarceration, particularly on women. And the fact that women who are incarcerated are as much victims as they are perpetrators of offences. Also, there's been a recognition of cognitive impairment as a relevant factor that requires special attention, although there is still a lack of screening for it. And, finally, there's been an increased acceptance that trauma and adverse childhood experiences cause lasting scars on people's psyches, and are associated with mental health disorders going forward as well as influencing offending trajectories. So those narratives have changed, but often the structural changes that should accompany that haven't."

The majority of the people Sullivan works with share something in common. They were always already vulnerable in that they lacked access to support. Often, in the early stages of developing a severe psychotic illness, you'll falter at school or work, and struggle to maintain relationships. Statistically, you'll most likely deal with the resulting emotional distress by self-medicating with drugs or alcohol. "The message of early intervention is that retaining people in education or work for as long as possible provides them with something to fall back on in the future. If you fall out of education, and are not employable from your teens, you have a very limited opportunity to participate in the benefits of society. Substance use complicates that, and worsens mental health, but is also associated with socio-economic deterioration. So all of the factors link together to lead to people being more marginalised." These problems are compounded by imprisonment, which untethers you from relationships, accommodation, treating clinicians. "So when you get out, like snakes and ladders, you're often way down the scale and you have to start again. It becomes very difficult to get back on your feet ... In some of the other states with higher Indigenous populations, the number of people from Indigenous communities who are in contact with the criminal justice system is just staggering. Whether that's because of the absence of opportunities to divert, particularly in remote communities, or the lack of infrastructure, it clearly means that people are being kicked in the guts repeatedly.

"I think there are islands of efforts to assist, but they're not necessarily joined up.

"As a point of philosophical pride in a civil society," Sullivan continues, "people with a mental health disorder should be treated in a mental health facility. I feel strongly that people with significant mental health disorders who have offended should be transferred from prison to a secure hospital and receive the therapeutic interventions which address their offending needs, as well as their mental health needs." This is not currently the case – when you consider that Thomas Embling currently has twenty beds for the entire male prison population, and that at least 40 per cent of Victoria's prisoners were assessed as having a mental health condition, you can understand why.

*

Despite the fact that mental illness is so prevalent that someone who has grappled with it personally has written this and is, probably, reading this, there are ethical reporting guidelines to ensure that harmful stereotypes are not perpetuated. That is why I will mention here, for the purposes of clarity, that most people with a mental illness have no history of violence. Given that, my final question for Sullivan is why the idea lives so prominently in the public discourse that "the mentally ill" are a population to fear.

"Historically, mad people were equated with raving beasts or with people who were less than human," he replies. "With the growth of civil rights discourse in the 1960s and '70s, I think people tried to invert that message and suggest that, in fact, people with mental health disorders were no more likely than others to commit offences. The evidence clearly indicates that people with severe mental health disorders, particularly when complicated by personality disorder or substance use, have significantly increased rates of violent offending. But that of course refers to individuals, not to the population as a whole." It's important, he continues, that you don't stigmatise or stereotype all people in a category, although there may be an increased prevalence. That prevalence, he points out, also reflects the failings of our community to provide adequately funded resources to offset that risk.

"It's hard sometimes to provide positive media about this," he says, as he gets ready to go to court. "The person goes on leave, goes to their job, returns on time. It's not a media story but it happens every day."

*

The sky is still gun-metal grey when I leave the hospital and walk over to the gate post where the asylum once stood. There, a dirty silver plaque reads:

> "It was not pleasant when walking quietly in the garden at eve, to be startled by the wild maniac laughter that came echoing down the river" – Lucy Anna Edgar (Merri Creek Aboriginal School) reflecting on the Yarra Bend Asylum. This location was chosen for the asylum as the Yarra River almost surrounded the area, providing excellent security. The asylum operated here between 1848 and 1925. At times over 1000 inmates were housed here and the asylum was almost a self-sufficient township. Unfortunately, conditions were poor and residents suffered hardship ...

Despite nearly a decade of passing this plaque on my run, I never realised it was there. I consider stopping some of those strolling with prams or dogs to ask if they've read it. But I swallow the question and get into the quiet of my car. Moments later, curving around the back of the hospital on my way home, the Italianate turret of the old Kew Lunatic Asylum rises like a lighthouse out of the waving treetops.

Perched on "a gentle eminence in a fertile and agreeable country," Kew Lunatic Asylum was one of the largest mental institutions in the country. A "magnificent asylum for the insane," it was a dark mirror in which Marvellous Melbourne could gaze at its benevolent image. The first public inquiry into its operation occurred in 1876, five years after it opened.

Patients slept in rows running down the lines of the building's two wings. Men to the right, women to the left. Less space was given to the women's wards, where the laundries and drying yards were located. The wards were further divided in the still-current human taxonomies of paying/pauper, manageable/refractory. Familiar too are their diagnoses: puerperal mania (postnatal depression), melancholia (depression), inebriation (alcoholism, addiction), dementia, delusional insanity (schizophrenia), epilepsy, idiocy (intellectual disability).

Initially, wards of the state, "difficult" children, and children with intellectual disability were housed with the adults at Kew. Then the Children's Cottages at Kew opened in 1887 as the Idiot Ward of Kew Asylum. As the technical term for severe intellectual disability, "idiot" would remain in legal and medical use for decades, based on Dr Henry Goddard's concept of mental age. In descending order of capacity: morons, imbeciles, idiots. "Moron" was the newest word: early-twentieth-century, meaning foolish, stupid. "Imbecile" was sixteenth-century English for weak or feeble. "Idiot" was the oldest label. It derived from the Greek *idios*, meaning "private" or "one's own"; that isolated place as necessary to the collective dream of the settlers and their descendants as it has been terrifying in their nightmares.

Closing in 1988, Kew Asylum was eventually developed into the Willsmere residential complex, which is currently marketed as "tranquil, serene and friendly living at its best"; "Willsmere – it's a great place to live!" A condition of the development permit was that a section of the building be maintained as a museum. A "fever tent" has been preserved, and a section of the "Female Paying Patients Ward." There is now a pool, a playground. The Willsmere residential development was officially opened in 1993 by Victorian premier Jeff Kennett, who – over the next year – presided over the rapid deinstitutionalisation of the state's inpatient facilities and the removal of those people into underfunded housing and under-resourced community services. Kennett would go on to found Beyond Blue in 2000, and was its chairman for seventeen years as it raised awareness of depression, anxiety and suicide prevention.

As you drive down the green stretch of the main drive, where old pine trees seem to sweep the sky, you wouldn't know that this is where Kew Cottages burnt to the ground in 1996 after years of safety warnings, the lungs of its adult residents filling with smoke as they ran, terrified, through the halls in their pyjamas.

Even before you understand the story it contains, the title of the Victorian ombudsman's 2018 report conveys all the understated horror of a Kafka story: *Investigation into the Imprisonment of a Woman Found Unfit to Stand Trial*. And in her devastating opening, Deborah Glass matched the master: "This is the saddest case I have investigated in my time as Ombudsman." She continued: "A 39-year-old woman spent over 18 months in prison, locked in her cell up to 23 hours a day, where she would scream with distress for hours on end. She had been charged with breaching an intervention order taken out by her family, who could not cope with her behaviour, and resisting police. This woman, whom we refer to as Rebecca, was found unfit to stand trial and not guilty because of mental impairment. She remained in prison simply because there was nowhere for her to go. Had she pleaded guilty to the offence, she would have been sentenced to serve less time than she ended up spending in prison."

Despite a lifelong history of behavioural difficulties, professionals couldn't agree on whether Rebecca had a mental illness or an intellectual disability. There was agreement that she required support but not on who was responsible for providing it. The changing diagnoses meant that "she fell into a service gap." "While agencies mostly followed procedure, and in some cases went beyond them in an attempt to provide support," Glass continued, "the State failed Rebecca."

This report exists because the Public Advocate, Colleen Pearce, raised concerns with the ombudsman about the imprisonment of Rebecca, who had become one of her clients. "We are guardian for a small group of people within the correctional system," Pearce tells me. "Generally, they are people on remand or found unfit to be tried. They have multiple disabilities. We find them in the criminal justice system, where they're detained for long periods of time when they otherwise might have been released, but they're not released because there are inadequate supports for them."

Pearce explains that these clients, with a complex presentation of their disabilities, have often been subjected to significant childhood trauma at home or in the child protection system. She points to another case, involving an Indigenous man with fetal alcohol syndrome and a moderate intellectual disability, who was held on remand for 543 days due to lack of accommodation after being found unfit to be tried. "They are deeply traumatised individuals and the challenging behaviours they exhibit can be an indication of the frustration of their inability to communicate their needs and their wants," she explains. Close and continuing relationships, especially with clinicians, are key to their treatment – the type of trauma-informed care that was emphasised by the Royal Commission. That's not what they reliably receive. Instead, Pearce says, the experience of being detained in the prison system – locked down for long periods of time for reasons they may be unable to understand – is itself "deeply traumatising."

"Having examined Rebecca's case, we wanted to find out if the problem was systemic," the ombudsman wrote. Glass's investigation demonstrated the case was not an isolated incident. How isolated, however, couldn't be said. No data is kept on how many people like Rebecca are in prison. No agency is responsible for tracking people deemed unfit to stand trial. The investigation revealed other stories like Rebecca's, which highlighted "both the trauma of incarceration on acutely vulnerable people, and the threat to community safety in failing to provide a safe and therapeutic alternative to prison." Around the country, in the absence of early and appropriate diagnosis, intervention and community-based supports, disadvantaged people with mental and cognitive disability, in particular Indigenous Australians, are being "systematically criminalised" – managed by, and entrenched in, the criminal justice system.

Rebecca and I were about the same age – thirty-nine – when the Public Advocate referred her case to the ombudsman. We enjoy some of the same things: music, looking at magazines generally and pictures of the royal family specifically, the beach, the world changing gradually on a long drive. It wouldn't matter, though, if we had nothing in common. It shouldn't. Though, given what was done to her in our name, her story eloquently demonstrates otherwise.

Rebecca's parents took her to a paediatrician at four years old because she was "different." She was referred for psychological and other assessments from the age of nine. She had "difficulties" with other students, and left school (like Eliza and Daylia) in Year 8. Into early adulthood, she had communicative difficulties and "behaviours of concern" – verbally abusing or assaulting carers, destroying property. This sometimes led to the police being called, which sometimes resulted in a decision to proceed with criminal charges.

Clinicians did not agree on Rebecca's diagnosis. From her teens and into her thirties, she was diagnosed with various mental health conditions, including possible personality disorders. At thirty-two, she was diagnosed with "pervasive developmental disorder not otherwise specified" and borderline intellectual function by the Victorian Dual Disability Service, which works with specialist mental health services to treat people with both a mental illness and a developmental disability. However, the Victorian Department of Health and Human Services disputed this diagnosis when it assessed Rebecca the following year. There was also disagreement about whether she had an intellectual disability. The Victorian *Disability Act* requires an intellectual disability to have been "manifest" before the age of eighteen. When Rebecca was tested at twelve, she recorded an IQ of eighty-four. This was above the threshold for intellectual disability – seventy or below. When she was tested again at the age of thirty-four, she recorded an IQ of sixty-five. However, she had missed the age cut-off.

The official diagnosis mattered because it determined the services available to her. Victoria's services for people with a mental impairment are divided into two streams. First, the mental health system provides services to people who have a treatable mental illness under the *Mental Health Act*. Second, the disability services system provides services to people with a disability under the *Disability Act*. These include intellectual disability, acquired brain injury and neurological impairments such as autism spectrum disorder. From her teens into her thirties, Rebecca received services through the mental health system. This included extended periods living in her local mental health service's acute care, secure extended care and community care units. However, her new diagnosis of pervasive developmental disorder and borderline intellectual function meant she was no longer eligible for those services. The area mental health service discharged her just before she turned thirty-five. The discharge notes refer to her "lack of an axis 1 psychiatric disorder," her unwillingness to engage with treatment and the wishes of Rebecca and her family. "It was decided that [Rebecca] should be discharged ... with her care being transferred to a GP. Her GP can refer her on to Disability Services if this is felt necessary in the future" – which, technically, she was by then too old to qualify for. The only place we had for Rebecca was in the gap.

"In terms of functional capacity to exist in the world and to operationalise her own interests, [she was] the most impaired person I've represented," Tim Marsh says of Rebecca, who was his client. "And she was deemed ineligible for disability services because she 'did not have a disability,' because in order to have a disability under the *Disability Act*, you need to have demonstrated evidence of it prior to the age of eighteen. Now, I don't know the circumstances of that IQ test, whether it was valid or reliable or repeatable, but that she was denied access to services because of something like that, when she was clearly unbelievably impaired, just goes to show you the type of sorting exercises that occur."

Rebecca's parents couldn't cope with her behaviour. In 2015, the Magistrates' Court issued a family violence intervention order that prevented Rebecca going within 200 metres of the family home. Aside from the fact that even mild changes can be devastating for someone with her diagnosis, it is unclear whether she had the capacity to understand the order in the first place. But assuming she did, I wonder what capacity she had to adapt to the reality of it. Even when it is a distressing place, it is near-impossible for the rest of us to integrate the cold fact that home is no longer home.

Despite the order, Rebecca kept returning. Her family would call the police; she would refuse to leave. One police statement describes her hiding under a blanket in a bedroom, curled into a ball. Police officers would lay hands on her, physically carry her from the house. On some occasions, officers took her to the local hospital. Other occasions resulted in charges. She was first remanded, for sixteen days, in mid-2015 after assaulting a staff member at a supported residential service. A fortnight later, she was imprisoned for breaching the intervention order, resisting police and other charges. She spent over five months there, although the prison transferred her to Thomas Embling Hospital for several weeks during that time. On her release from prison, she was given two nights' crisis accommodation in a hotel. Five weeks later, she was imprisoned again, for thirteen days, for breaching the intervention order and resisting police. On her release, the prison was unable to find crisis accommodation, so she was given public transport tickets and "limited transport assistance." She refused to get dressed, refused to leave her cell. Had to be "taken out to freedom" by emergency response group officers.

A fortnight later, she was in prison again, for twelve days, for breaching the intervention order and related charges. There are no records showing where she went when she was released, but she returned home a week later. After several days, her parents called the police following an argument. She was, yet again, charged with breaching the intervention order and resisting police. They took her to the local station, where a medical officer found her unfit to be interviewed. Less than a fortnight after she left prison, she was remanded again. The fifth time in nine months. This time she would stay for over eighteen months. "You tell me where the criminality is in her conduct," Marsh says, two years later. "That's a service failure issue. She spent eighteen months on remand because of service failure, not because she was a bad person."

It is an irony that Dame Phyllis Frost, for whom the only prison in Victoria that holds women on remand is named, was known for her "enormous capacity to get things done" and "shear through red tape." According to the Australian Women's Register: "Her Christian philosophy of love your neighbour and treat others as you would like to be treated, together with the belief that it is only in helping others that the human spirit can achieve happiness and rest, underpinned her work." In this building bearing Frost's name, Rebecca, in her sorrow and desperation, lost half her bodyweight.

The men's prison system in Victoria has a specialist unit for intellectually disabled prisoners. There is no equivalent in the women's system. Women who cannot be housed in mainstream units because of "behaviours of concern" have two options. The first is a management unit which goes by the curious name of Swan 2. Swan 2 is a prison within a prison, where people punished for disciplinary offences are routinely locked in their cells for twenty-two to twenty-three hours a day in conditions the Ombudsman described elsewhere as "bleak." The second option is the mental health unit, called Marrmak, where prison officers work alongside Forensicare clinicians who provide specialist care for women with serious psychiatric conditions. These clinicians do not necessarily have training in treating people with intellectual disabilities. Correctional officers certainly don't have that training. Prison is not a disability setting.

On entry, Rebecca presented as extremely unwell to staff who were, by now, familiar with her. Records of her first days note she refused food. She was yelling, crying, asking for her father.

After spending her first nights in the medical centre, Rebecca was moved to Swan 2 "to allow ongoing psych[iatric] and medical assessment and observation." Prison officers described her behaviour as "erratic" and prisoners verbally abused her. After three weeks in the management unit, Corrections Victoria moved Rebecca to Marrmak. When interviewed by the ombudsman, the Forensicare psychiatrist at Marrmak described the management unit as unsuitable for people like Rebecca, saying that their mental state deteriorates there, that it's a downward spiral. While Marrmak is better, in that it has a psychologist and can engage other supports, it is also not designed for people with intellectual disabilities or developmental disorders.

When Rebecca arrived at the prison, she did not have funding under the National Disability Insurance Scheme or an appointed legal guardian. Forensicare applied to enrol Rebecca in the NDIS. It also applied to the Victorian Civil and Administrative Tribunal to appoint a legal guardian for her. There was less progress, however, by all parties concerned, in securing accommodation or services so that Rebecca could leave prison. She was initially placed in Marrmak to ensure that she did not become a long-term "management" prisoner in the disciplinary unit. However, in Marrmak, she was also locked in her cell for twenty-two to twenty-three hours a day. The International Standards for the Treatment of Prisoners define solitary confinement as confinement for twenty-two hours or more a day without meaningful human contact. The effects on the health of prisoners include anxiety, depression and psychosis. People with impaired functioning are especially at risk. In November 2016, a prison officer noted that Rebecca was deteriorating.

There was initial confusion about whether Rebecca's parents could contact her because of their intervention orders against Rebecca. In January 2017, a prison officer recorded that her parents had been calling but were denied permission to speak with her, and that the prison had withheld a Christmas card from her mother. The officer wrote, "[Rebecca] thinks her parents passed away and we are hiding it from her." After the officer raised this issue within the unit, the prison appears to have clarified the situation, because Rebecca began having telephone calls with her father, as well as some visits.

Bringing to mind things hidden or dirty or in need of daylight, the time a prisoner spends outside their cell is referred to as an "airing." Initially, Rebecca was allowed a minimum of one one-hour airing a day. In early 2017, an external psychologist found that this urgently needed to be increased. In April 2017, an officer noted she had been crying after her airing. "I think she is very lonely and needs more interaction. I spoke with [the Forensicare nurses] about [Rebecca's] vocabulary and mental health as I have noticed it has deteriorated in the past 12 months." Later that month, the same officer wrote, "I have major concerns that [Rebecca's] health is deteriorating." In mid-May, the prison started giving her a second one-hour airing. For the rest of the time, she remained in her cell, sometimes soothing herself by combing her hair.

The ombudsman found that prison officers in Marrmak "tried to provide meaningful human contact for Rebecca when she was out of her cell, although her disabilities made this challenging." For the first few months, an officer explained, when they opened her door, Rebecca would "stay in her cell and get in the bottom of the shower and hold on to her head and scream constantly, just scream." On one occasion, a prison officer wrote: "Rebecca sounds like the exorcist over the intercom as she continues to spit and scream like a scene from a horror movie." It was noted that she sometimes insulted other women in the unit, that her screaming kept them awake at night, that they were given earplugs to block out the noise. The other prisoners were locked down during Rebecca's airings; more time out of her cell meant less time for them.

Initially, she required support for her personal care: getting dressed, using sanitary items, using toilet paper. She was scared of the shower. A Marrmak officer said that it was "like looking after a kid." She would sometimes refuse food, and lost over fifty kilograms in the first seven months. At the time, there was no formal system for providing personal care support to prisoners with disabilities. Prison officers provided this support to her on their own initiative – mopping her floors, stripping her bed, doing her laundry. Officers and Forensicare staff spent time encouraging her to eat and to shower. One officer said that she sometimes gave Rebecca her dinner on a plate, with proper cutlery, and ate with her so Rebecca had someone to talk to over the dinner table.

Over time, Rebecca started to come out and talk with the officers. Prison records describe Forensicare's occupational therapist and other staff sometimes involving her in activities such as cooking. On other occasions, she verbally abused or spat at officers, tipped over furniture during her airings, threw food and other objects. She was sent back to Swan 2 for two days in September 2016 for spitting at officers, and for fourteen days in June 2017 for assaulting an officer. She was subject to a "handcuff regime" whenever she was out of her cell. After her time in Swan 2, her hygiene deteriorated.

An officer helped Rebecca budget her prison allowance so she could purchase food and personal items. She was given magazines for a time, but that ceased because she would tear them up and block the toilet. If there was enough toilet paper, she would also use it to block the toilet. She broke the toilet seat and then it was removed from her cell. Her guardian questioned the prison's response, explaining that Rebecca was bored, stating, "I'd be [breaking things] if I was locked in a cell for twenty-four hours."

Corrections Victoria's *Sentence Management Manual* requires a behavioural management plan when separation is used to manage the challenging behaviour of prisoners with cognitive impairment. The plan should be developed by a disability clinician and reviewed weekly, lockdown should be part of a staged process and a last option, it should only be used for up to four hours in any day, and prisoners can only be locked down on three consecutive days without a formal review. Instead, the versions of Rebecca's intensive case management plan were prepared by prison officers and provided for her to be locked down for twenty-two to twenty-three hours a day over an extended period.

Forensicare had given Rebecca a weighted toy cat in September 2016, weighted items being a calming sensory tool and not only for those with autism (think of your doona, the effect of a hand on your hand, and why being held causes a baby's heart rate to slow down). Prison officers gave her a teddy bear in November 2016. Other items permitted in her cell as of August 2017: "one book or magazine issued and swapped only at mealtimes (and removed if misused), toiletries, writing pad. 1 × Flexi Pen. Puzzle/word searches (95 pages per day, as per daily request only). 1 × pet therapy cat (white). 1 × black and white pillowcase (Mary had a little lamb). 1 × toilet roll – if misused, to be replace [sic] with 15 sheets of toilet paper (Staff be mindful, Prisoner will use excessive amounts of TP and clothing items). Prison issue clothing. Bedding pack. One comb (DO NOT REMOVE UNLESS APPROVED BY UNIT SPO/SUP), No sharps (Tweezers, nail clippers, plastic cutlery or plastic containers)."

I think of Rebecca, exhausted, diminished, combing her hair like a banshee. How she, too, was reduced in her pain to just her cry, a keening omni-directional scream with a message for all of us.

*

Why was there nowhere for Rebecca? Service gaps. Stand-offs. Legislative failures. The answer restates the question. There have been many reviews of secure therapeutic facilities over the years, all of which highlighted the acute shortage of beds, particularly for women with disabilities. Everyone involved with Rebecca's situation acknowledged it was unacceptable. Forensicare wrote to the Magistrates' Court after Rebecca had been in prison for around two months, asking it to adjourn her case for eight to ten weeks so that the agencies involved could put a plan in place. It took another sixteen and a half months and many more court hearings before a solution was found.

Like psychologists and psychiatrists and doctors and sociologists and writers and readers, bureaucrats impose categories for use as perceptual shorthand on the otherwise undifferentiated contents of reality. But if the objective is knowledge – that is, proximity – labels only go so far before they exacerbate distance. What is known as "the mental health system," for example, is really just billions of human interactions. And that is where the problems lie.

The first meeting of agencies to discuss Rebecca's situation was held in June 2016. There would be at least seventeen such meetings. Minutes show these meetings were highly populated and often included senior profes-sionals. One meeting had eighteen people. Another meeting had so many people in the room there were almost two layers of chairs around the table. They agreed to look for interim housing so Rebecca could leave prison, and options for supported accommodation so she could ultimately return to the community. The was no single person or agency responsible for helping people such as Rebecca, who fall outside the standard remit of mental health and disability services, and it wasn't clear who exactly was accountable for securing housing. "The action plans from case conference meetings between July and October 2016 list the 'lead agency' for deter-mining accommodation options as 'All,'" Glass noted. Everyone was responsible, so no one was responsible.

Forensicare could not accept Rebecca at Thomas Embling because she did not have a treatable mental illness. Her diagnosis – pervasive developmental disorder – is defined as a permanent disability. Given that, DHHS said Rebecca also could not be treated in an acute inpatient unit, because it would have represented a breach of her human rights. Disability services, however, could not provide a solution. There are two secure accommodation options for people with disabilities under the *Crimes (Mental Impairment and Unfitness to Be Tried) Act*. The first is an all-male facility which houses sex offenders. The second is the Long-Term Rehabilitation Program, a five-bed unit in Bundoora. DHHS advised that admission is limited to people with intellectual disabilities. Due to the timing of her diagnosis, Rebecca did not satisfy the legislative definition. The Forensicare psychiatrist tried to find an appropriate residential disability service for people with autism spectrum disorders in Victoria; "unfortunately there are none."

The Multiple and Complex Needs Initiative (MACNI) is a specialist program managed by DHHS for people with combinations of mental illness, substance dependence, intellectual impairment or acquired brain injury who pose a risk to themselves or others. The MACNI program was willing to assist Rebecca, even though she did not meet its criteria. MACNI, however, does not provide accommodation. Although mental health services, disability services and MACNI fall under a single department, the issues were not resolved. The ombudsman heard that DHHS has become more "siloed" because of restructuring; that when you have more silos, people become more "precious" and the criteria get tougher. Victoria's Chief Psychiatrist told the ombudsman that he didn't have the feeling any individual or service sector was to blame for the situation, that it was just the gaps: "Even with the willingness of people to come together, there were some structural, systemic challenges for us getting the solution."

Marsh described the experience of attending one of these meetings differently. How he watched people go around the table metaphorically, and in some cases literally, pointing the finger at each other. "Eventually I had to say, 'She's not staying here forever. She's going to come out and this case is in front of a judge who will not hesitate to require you to come to court and explain why you're not doing anything.'"

In June 2017, a MACNI assessment panel formally agreed to provide some support for Rebecca. The next day, MACNI identified a viable DHHS-owned house. In August 2017, after a number of difficulties and delays, the National Disability Insurance Agency approved an NDIS plan for Rebecca with over $1.3 million in funding. It paid for two care workers to support Rebecca around the clock. The OPA guardian said, in her opinion, Rebecca's plan was so expensive because prison had made her behaviour worse and she became more of a risk.

"It's concerning," Marsh told the court on the day of Rebecca's release, "that somebody who is as acutely vulnerable as [Rebecca] could nevertheless spend eighteen months in custody on matters which would have been unlikely to attract a custodial sentence had she been able to plead guilty to them in the first place." It was Taft, again, on the bench – a judge who happened to have a particular interest in disability and in holding administrative agencies responsible for their failures. In endorsing Marsh's remarks, Taft stated that the fact Rebecca had been in custody for so long, "reflects very poorly on the criminal justice system and on the welfare system."

The ombudsman would find that Rebecca's human rights had been breached. That her case highlights "a lack of suitable options for people with disabilities and high-risk behaviours in Victoria," which the state is responsible for providing. In her most recent report, she wrote that "it is an indictment on our claim to be a just society that [Rebecca's] case was far from unique," and that like cases continue to be reported. "While I am pleased the Minister has accepted my recommendation that the State invest in therapeutic alternatives to prison, we have not yet seen meaningful progress."

Colleen Pearce, the Public Advocate, tells me that Rebecca is doing well. The supported accommodation secured for her in the community "ultimately did not prove successful," so she was admitted to a specialist secure hospital unit, where her disruptive behaviours improved and where she is working with a therapeutic team towards a goal of returning to reside in the community. In addition to a dearth of skilled service providers, housing remains the key issue for people with complex needs like Rebecca. Pearce explains that most people in that category have to rent, leaving them without certain protections. "They can be evicted, outside of the safeguarding of *Residential Tenancies Act*, and also you're not entitled to visits from community visitors," she says.

This is the first I've heard of "community visitors." There are 650 of them. Pearce calls them "human rights volunteers" and "the eyes and ears of the community." "They're volunteers who work with my office, empowered under legislation to visit disability houses, acute mental health services and supported residential services," she explains. "They go in to monitor the wellbeing and human rights of people in closed environments. One of the key safeguards that Victoria has for people in those settings is community visitors."

I ask Pearce whether this would ideally be a paid position. "No," she replies, "we're happy with them being volunteers because in Victoria they're part of the social capital of the state. They volunteer to give their time to protect and promote the rights of people with disability, and they have the support of my office. They are not paid professionals and they are utterly independent."

My feeling about this remains one of profound ambivalence. On the one hand, a personal commitment to the care of vulnerable people is the type of behaviour without which a society cannot flourish. On the other hand, ensuring the protection of human rights in closed, state-regulated environments is not a responsibility government can devolve to private citizens. This is particularly relevant given that people with disability in Australia are at a significantly greater risk of experiencing physical and sexual violence than those without disability. Women with an intellectual or psychological disability are nearly three times more likely than women with a physical disability to experience violence.

Nationally, the number of supported housing places is less than half of what is required to accommodate individuals with disabilities or severe mental illness who are at significant risk of housing instability. In the absence of effective oversight, and with annual NDIS funding packages which can be worth over $1 million, those who require supported residential services are vulnerable to exploitation. Originally established in the 1970s, to care for the elderly, supported residential services became the default option for people with mental illness left homeless by the underfunded deinstitutionalisation of mental health facilities in the mid-1990s. About 4000 Victorians with a disability and/or mental illness live in 117 supported residential homes – facilities that are privately owned but state-regulated. Hambleton House, in one of Melbourne's wealthiest neighbourhoods, was one of them. In 2020, its residents were evacuated after squalid conditions were discovered when fifteen of its twenty-eight residents tested positive for Covid-19. Though the state government closed the facility and relocated its residents, the Public Advocate had raised serious concerns about Hambleton House for years.

"In the community we probably had trust that a place like Hambleton House would be well regulated," someone who lived nearby told *The Age*. "In a country like ours, how could it possibly not be?" Their shock echoed that in the Oakden Review, the 2017 inquiry into "deplorable" practices at the Oakden Older Persons Mental Health Service in South Australia: "How could Oakden exist in some parallel world, unable to embrace modern patterns of care?" Perhaps, however, the biggest shock of all is that there are no parallel worlds, just this one. No institutions, just individuals. No them, just us. Sontag said it: "Someone who is perennially surprised that depravity exists, who continues to feel disillusioned (even incredulous) when confronted with evidence of what humans are capable of inflicting in the way of gruesome, hands-on cruelties upon other humans, has not reached moral or psychological adulthood. No one after a certain age has the right to this kind of innocence, of superficiality, to this degree of ignorance or amnesia."

"It seems generally true that members of a social category may strongly support a standard of judgment that they and others agree does not apply directly to them."

—Erving Goffman, *Stigma*

The current mess has arrived right on time. The Victorian Royal Commission pointed out that the Victorian government has known "for at least a decade" about the "challenges" posed by the mental health system. The Department of Health's 2009 mental health strategy, for example, stated that action was needed "not only to address the current needs of the Victorian population but to plan for the projected numbers of people likely to be seeking help for mental health problems in ten years' time." The Royal Commission's 2019 report quoted Simon Straface, now Chief Adviser of Mental Health Reform Victoria:

The system is achieving exactly the results it was set up to achieve, every time a decision was made to take funding out, without keeping track of its impact on patients and their families. It is achieving the results it was set up for, every time decisions were made to fragment the system further by introducing elements that linked poorly with one another ... every time we ... turned a blind eye to deteriorating hospitals, the substandard accommodation, the homelessness, the poverty and the violence that is all too common an experience for people with severe mental illness ... We all have a hand in where we are today.

The problem is not unique to Victoria. In a 1981 volume of the *Australian and New Zealand Journal of Psychiatry*, there appeared an article by a psychologist named Peter Wells titled "The Need for Mental Health Services for Adolescents in the Hunter Region." "A sample of disturbed youngsters making demands on agencies in the City of Newcastle and on community health teams and school guidance in the rest of the Region suggests that during November 1980 only about one in 20 of those in need were receiving help from these agencies," Wells wrote. "Eighty-five percent involved major family issues. Of those receiving help, at least 40 percent would have been referred to an adolescent mental health service, had there been one. Of the alternatives that had to be used, about 75 percent were estimated to have been less than adequate."

Forty years later, Adrian Plaskett, a GP who has worked in the Hunter Region since 1999, will write, in response to *The Guardian*'s reader call-out about the mental health system, that the area Headspace – the mental health service for young people – has a four-month waitlist. Plaskett described alarming trends. He wrote that when he started as a GP, he had a relationship with clinicians at the local mental health service that did outreach for severely ill people. He could ring them directly and together they could organise a call-out to a patient's home, where, if necessary, a psychiatry registrar, an ambulance and a police officer would attend and make decisions about the best course of action. Now he has no direct way of contacting the local mental health team; his calls go to a statewide 1800 number. Without a community outreach service, he explained, people tend to go further into crisis until the police are called. "I imagine this service is far cheaper to run, but it means problems are more likely to get out of control before they are dealt with." He is no longer informed about patients who are placed on the "acute list," nor actively involved with local mental health services. After the immediate crisis passes, there is no ongoing follow-up with a clinician who knows them and has a relationship with them. "In general people with severe mental illness such as schizophrenia in Newcastle who are stable do not have any ongoing contact with a psychiatrist (unless they have money)," he wrote.

The community health centres which had provided cognitive behavioural therapy for low-income patients with severe but not acutely life-threatening illness no longer exist. Headspace, its closest replacement, serves young people only and is at capacity. This, Plaskett wrote, is one of the reasons there is a high rate of antidepressant prescription for mild mental illness that would be better treated in the young with talking therapy; "It's because GPs and drugs are far easier to access than psychologists and therapy." Many cannot afford to pay the gap between their Medicare mental health plan and private psychology fees. Moreover, while the limited number of sessions are helpful for problems such as grief or mild anxiety, "patients with severe and ongoing problems like psychotic illnesses, victims of childhood sexual abuse (of which there are huge numbers), entrenched personality disorders, perpetrators of domestic violence, dual and complex diagnoses between drugs and mental health, and so on, for these people five sessions at $60 or $80 a pop are just not going to help." Since Plaskett wrote his article, you can now claim up to twenty sessions with a mental health professional each year. Getting into a bulk-billed local psychology practice can be difficult. For patients who go private, Medicare usually covers only part of that cost. Health professionals set their own fees and the Australian Psychological Society's recommended fee for a standard consultation is currently $267. That is more than half the average national weekly rent for a house or a unit. Even with the rebate, twenty sessions can work out to be prohibitively priced for many.

Rural and regional GPs from around the nation echo Plaskett's concern that despite there being more psychiatrists than cardiologists in Australia, there is a chronic undersupply of the former in the communities these GPs serve. Psychiatrists tend to be concentrated in large metropolitan centres and focus on private patients. "Even in a city the size of Newcastle," Plaskett wrote, "I have given up trying to get patients to see a psychiatrist here as their books are closed or their prices are so expensive that they have clearly made a decision to only serve the wealthy."

After he finishes administering Covid-19 vaccines, Plaskett, still in scrubs, hops in his car to chat with me on Zoom. "What a GP is an expert in is perhaps the local community," he says. "You get to know people quite well over the years. That's not just me, it's the whole practice milieu." I will learn that, as far as interview subjects go, he is a rara avis. He has over twenty years of first-hand experience and is more interested in conveying and learning information than in what Goffman called "impression management."

When it comes to access to mental health treatment, Plaskett says much depends on the illness. "People with chronic schizophrenia, where they tick the boxes, have benefited greatly from the NDIS." If chronically ill people cannot get onto that pathway, however, they are at loose ends. "The other group is people who have personality problems – BPD or violent offenders – they require a lot of work to overcome these problems and that's not really available.

"Sarah, I'm a person who writes quite a lot of letters," Plaskett replies, with a wry smile, when I ask why he felt called to write his letter to *The Guardian*. "I write to politicians, mainly about climate change – that's the biggest public health emergency that we seem to be ignoring, but that's another story. So it was not unusual for me to write that thing. I'm not an expert in mental health, but if they'd been talking about joint replacement surgery, I could've written exactly the same thing. I think the changes that have occurred in the mental health system are not dissimilar to changes that have occurred in other aspects of the health system, and indeed changes that have occurred in society at large.

"I think there's been a general move towards a more individualistic, self-funded mode of living that's really been reflected across society. It goes back, I reckon, to around the time of Thatcher, the mid-'80s. There was this general movement into this view that capitalism was the way to go and that's been reflected in all areas of society. Now, in the health system in Australia, if you're not privately insured, it just takes a long time.

"Say you've got a bad knee – you're a 75-year-old with an osteoarthritic knee. I can get you a knee replacement within two months if you're in the private system. If you're in the public system, you're waiting a year for your appointment, and another year before surgery. That's just too long. It's so long that in that time all sorts of things start to happen – you lose your mobility, you start to get depressed, you get hooked on opiate drugs.

It's this cascade of consequences. In Newcastle, that's certainly the case with orthopaedic surgery; neurology; urology; ophthalmology; ear, nose and throat; and psychiatry.

"So I don't see it as anything that's unique to mental health, this difference between people who are financially secure and in the private system versus people who are not so financially secure and in the public system. When I started work twenty years ago, I could genuinely say to people, 'Private, public doesn't make any difference.' Famously, Paul Keating was not privately insured."

Plaskett does have a caveat that, when it comes to our health system, most other countries would happily trade places with us. And yet, from what he is describing, that appears to say more about the woeful state of medical provision elsewhere than it does about the excellence of our systems. He recounts how he took part in a gynaecology redesign project to make public clinics more user-friendly. "It was a room full of women, and I asked the question, 'Who here has used the clinic?' The only person who had actually used the public hospital clinic that they were designing was the Aboriginal liaison officer. Everyone else had private health. It's being used by people who don't have much resources and it's being designed by people who don't use it. In mental health, that's true as well."

This disconnect is important. In *The Guardian*, Plaskett observed a "general increase in awareness of mental health as a personal illness." In counterpoint, his motivation for writing that piece was to highlight the social determinants of mental health. "The truth is that while many mental illnesses are unpredictable and can strike anyone," he wrote, "there are also very real societal drivers of mental illness. Placing all the emphasis on the individual with programs like R U OK? allows the government to ignore the drivers of mental illness which are well known and well documented." He lists some: poverty, homelessness or insecure housing, powerlessness, lack of quality education, a feeling of hopelessness leading to drug use, lack of parenting support, disruptive and chaotic childhood without options for safety.

"We all break eventually given enough stress (as evidenced by senior politicians going off on stress leave in response to difficult circumstances at work despite their well-paid and supported environment. You don't get the option of 'stress leave' if you are stuck in an abusive relationship with no other housing option.)" Reading that, I thought of how society, like the psyche, is dissociable; made up of parts that can act in concert or be split off. We still discuss "the mental health system" as though it is independent of, or severable from, other systems. This is in my mind when I ask Plaskett why he reckons we have absolved ourselves, and our politicians, of the responsibility for properly investing in mental healthcare for so long.

"I think the answer is that there's this narrative – what does ScoMo say? – 'If you have a go, you get a go.' That's a highly American view of the world: the Wild West, the self-made person, 'if you just try hard enough …' That's really changed over the last forty or fifty years, with the fall of communism and the belief that the market is all there is, that we're rational creatures and if we make society that way then eventually it's going to be better for everybody. It's a form of trickle-down economics and everyone's bought into that belief – that if there's enough prosperity in society, then inevitably these webs of care will just appear, rather than be something that needs to be consciously constructed, as they were originally."

Plaskett mentions his wife, a housing researcher, and what he has learnt from her. "Our social welfare system in Australia was designed in the Second World War. As I understand it, at the height of the war when the bombs were falling on Darwin, the government designed a social welfare state. It was fought for. And that's been collectively forgotten. Most people seem to believe if you try harder, things are going to go alright." He looks ahead for a beat, the planes of his thin face stark against the window behind him, which is full of the blue sky.

"Ignore words and look at outcomes. For the health system, have a think about areas that work really well. Emergency – you have a car accident, you have a heart attack – we have extraordinarily good outcomes in

Australia. Intensive care — does a wonderful job. Any sort of emergency surgery — public health is great. Cancer is pretty good — my sister had breast cancer last year and it all went pretty smoothly. And then you ask yourself: what are the parts of the hospital that the middle class uses? There it is. What are the parts of the hospital that poorer people use? There it is. So the system is working as intended. If you look at the outcomes of the system, you'd say it is a system designed to maintain inequality and treat people with money.

"It's the same with the education system. That's just obvious to anyone who looks at it. As a doctor, my kids went to the local public selective school. It's great. If you send your kids to the local school at the housing commission, you're going to have first-year-out teachers who probably don't want to be there. Just look at the outcomes and you see systems are functioning as intended. It's a bit of a worry." This is what he had referred to, in his *Guardian* piece, when he wrote that the deterioration of our mental health services is just one aspect of "the general hollowing-out of the institutions of the state."

Earlier in the morning, Naomi Osaka was in the news for withdrawing from Wimbledon for mental health reasons. "On the one hand, you could say, whatever mental illness she's got, she copes with it magnificently," Plaskett says. "Yet in her mind, that's not the case. There's plenty of successful, outwardly coping people who've committed suicide. That's the double standard writ large: all these organisations saying we're so supportive but when push comes to shove, 'Well, actually it's your job to put up with it.'"

I ask whether he considers himself an optimist, and comment that he must be, given the hope for change at the heart of his letters.

"You've got to hope that we ..." He trails off, takes a breath, the bright day surrounding him. "I think humans essentially are a collective species, so you've got to hope that in the end problem-solving will triumph over divisiveness. You've got to do something, don't you? Really, it's a self-help thing. I've done a lot of learning about the branch of mental health called acceptance and commitment therapy. Part of that is trying to get in touch with your values and live life according to your values. Part of mine is to not be part of a system that enhances inequality. And I am. Over the last twenty years I've been part of a system that doesn't treat the poor well, it enhances the inequality between Indigenous people and others. The system as a whole is not something that's improving. And that's uncomfortable. So, personally, to try to feel better about that, I set aside some time each week to try to do something useful such as getting the message out there, or doing my little podcast, or handing out how-to-vote cards. It's not like it's altruistic; all these things are a mixture of making oneself feel better about the world. So that's why I do these things."

*

"The thing about GPs," Plaskett told me, "is we're quite a diverse group." I speak with many GPs, all of whom have at least ten years' experience in regional or rural practice. They've worked in mining towns and farming towns, in Far North Queensland and Western Tasmania and Eastern Victoria, the Northern Territory and the Kimberley. And while they were indeed a diverse group, they described similar things all over the country.

The Royal Commission found that GPs, along with police and emergency departments, are the frontline – and often the entirety – of mental healthcare in Victoria. The federal Productivity Commission found that GPs are likely to remain a dominant provider of mental healthcare services. The majority of their patients with mental health issues present with high prevalence conditions such as depression, anxiety, PTSD. A smaller number deal with psychotic illness. All the doctors expressed deep concerns about the current mental healthcare system. First, like Plaskett, they described a dearth of mental health support services, chronic workforce shortages in the area of mental health specifically and a lack of adequate communication between existing services and primary care physicians. "The referral process is – to be charitable – fairly broken," one said. This leaves their patients who need urgent help with very few options.

As another GP put it: "the purpose of mental health triage is to keep people away." "The best way," another said, "is to wait until after-hours and get to the hospital, which is an awful, cop-out way to do it, particularly for younger people. For adolescents it's a real struggle to find services." The Royal Commission estimated that in 2019–20, the system responded to less than one-third of the estimated demand for community mental health services across all age groups.

Professor Dennis Pashen, who speaks with me from Tasmania, has forty years' experience in rural and remote practice around the country. "The problems we have are access for the patients for support services. And that's universal," he explains.

"Where you've got a lack of access to support structures, patients tend to use their own initiative and either use alcohol or other drugs. The same issues exist everywhere. There's always been a conflict between mental health services and drug and alcohol services, and there's a lot of blame-shifting. Someone who has a significant self-medication issue with alcohol for their chronic, ongoing depression – they tend to be flicked past, and end up just getting dropped. They fall through that big gap in services.

"We tend, on the west coast of Tasmania, to get people brought in by relatives or police in a crisis. They tend to be transferred to the tertiary institution, assessed in the emergency department. They often end up discharged and back out on the street or admitted to the care unit, which is understaffed, as usual. There are no easy answers and I don't think anyone's had an answer so far.

"It's been a bit of a bugbear of mine that no one seems to accept responsibility. The government investment in mental health services has been minimal; even though they talk about it, the effectiveness has been minimal. The different state legislation in mental health has always been a problem. Each state has its own requirements, they're often complex and pretty unworkable."

Another concern the doctors had in common was the stress of trying to do their job to the best of their ability while they are overburdened by demand and the practice model only has so much flexibility. Again, Pashen: "Most practices run on about 40-plus per cent cost. Say if the doctor charges the bulk billing rate, 40 per cent goes to costs of the practice. If you're seeing someone for an hour, that's really not a cost-effective way of doing it. A lot of the big corporates – six-minute medicine – that's the most cost-effective way to get the turnover. And you can't do much in the mental health area in six minutes.

"We do double bookings, we'll see a patient and have them come back for a mental healthcare plan, which takes at least half an hour. We'll do the mental health assessment, then the mental healthcare plan, then we'll write the referral if needed and then we review them in six months. But in the meantime, the acute stuff usually re-presents either to the general practice or to the emergency department. It's a messy system, but continuity of care is really important. We don't get a lot of feedback in the meantime from the psychologists, we get some back from the public system – usually it's a 'discharge back into your care.'

"There's a reluctance with a lot of doctors working in rural and in metropolitan areas to take on the burden of ongoing continuous care. We have in our organisation employed doctors who have mental health as a focus of their clinical expertise, particularly suited to some of our communities where we've had a lot of mental health issues. These people usually don't last long because of the stress on them, the lack of supports they have personally … They have poor earnings because of the nature of billings within the system.

"There's no system that actually remunerates people who do the hard yards in mental health. It's really hard to treat mental health in general practice without the appropriate remuneration. Doesn't stop any of us doing it, but it is a disincentive [considering] the fullness of the need that's required within the community."

Mental healthcare is, intractably, time-intensive. It is also, to an enormous degree, relational. As one GP put it, "You can't delegate it very well. The holy grail of mental health at the moment is scalability – things you can do en masse rather than having one person spend an hour with one other person." This is also a serious issue for psychiatrists and psychologists, especially given that Medicare is oriented towards rewarding procedures, rather than therapy. But certain things require a human scale — attention and consistency over time is fundamental to the process. We can fund a model that better accommodates that reality, or not. One way or another, though — as Tim Marsh put it — we will pay for it.

*

Another concern voiced by the doctors I spoke with was the stigma of mental illness, particularly among men. You can start to see the scale of its impact when you consider, as one GP put it, that "most of men's health is heart disease and mental health."

Sarah Chalmers, who has practised in Townsville and the Northern Territory, is on the steering committee guiding the development of the National Stigma and Discrimination Reduction Strategy. She says that middle-aged male patients often present with physical issues — insomnia, memory issues, short tempers — and have to be gently told it's actually an issue with their mental health. Some are relieved to find it's treatable. Others are "very distressed" by the diagnosis; "they think you're insulting them." "With depression and anxiety," she explains, "I say to people who aren't really accepting of their own illness, 'You wouldn't be embarrassed by having diabetes. They don't have enough insulin, you don't have enough neurotransmitter.' With severe mental health, people will say, 'Oh, they can't help that,' but the social stigma is that those are people who can't cope, they're not resilient. And in an Australian culture, that's not cool. You cannot advertise your weakness.

"In the remote Northern Territory, we're all told that we're 'misfits, missionaries, or mercenaries,'" she says. "In the old days in the territories there were lots of troubled people running away from things. It's a good reason to go to places like that because you're surrounded by other people and you protect yourself; you don't ask them questions and they don't ask you questions, and you drink alcohol to dull your emotions and you shoot pigs, that's how they manage. They come in and ask, 'What's wrong with me?' You tell them mental health is a significant part of it. They're insulted you've called them crazy and then they build another little wall around themselves to ensure that they never make themselves vulnerable again."

It reminded me of Pashen's answer when I asked about stigma. "Australia's always had a bit of an attitude of 'She'll be right, mate.' 'Toughen up, girl.' 'You're a big boy now, you'll get over it.' Male culture is certainly rampant in rural areas," he said. "You know the classic story of the tough cattle-man – drinks to sedate himself and cover his depression, ends up shooting himself in the shed when no one's looking. The warning signs have been there and not been dealt with. We've always had this attitude."

> For Indigenous peoples, health itself is not understood as the con-
> cept often assumed by non-Indigenous people, rather it ... connects
> the health of an Indigenous individual to the health of their family,
> kin, community, and their connection to country, culture, spiritual-
> ity and ancestry.
>
> —Aboriginal and Torres Strait Islander Suicide Prevention
> Evaluation Project, "Solutions that work: What the evidence
> and our people tell us" (2016)

At a macro level, stigma reproduces social inequalities through the main-
tenance of group hierarchies. At a micro level, it is life-constricting, and
can be life-threatening. And like any other state-sanctioned violence, its
permissions spread.

Socially reviled attributes – whether racial or ethnic or religious or sexual
or physical or mental or behavioural – are fungible. There is nothing inherently discreditable about them. To understand stigma, Goffman was clear that
"a language of relationships, not attributes, is really needed." Stigma, in other
words, is not located in the Stigmatised or the Normal, but in the space
between them. "In the perpetual tally of Darwinian status encounters that
comprise Goffmanian social life," Rosemary Garland-Thompson wrote in
Disability Studies Quarterly, you come to the truth "that the normal have at best a
'shaky' advantage." Goffman was clear that even "the most fortunate Normal
is likely to have his half hidden failing, and for every little failing there is a
social occasion when it will loom large, creating a shameful gap between virtual and actual social identity." Normal is a performance, as specious as any
other externally assigned identity. There are, then, no true Normals: "the occa-
sionally precarious and the constantly precarious form a single continuum."
More than this, though: "The stigmatised and the normal are part of each
other; if one can prove vulnerable, it must be expected that the other can, too."

Much of what operates as vulnerability in Australia today started off as normal human variation (in, for example, race, sexuality, biology or geography) before it was socially converted into disadvantage. "Social exclusion and disadvantage are strongly associated with mental ill-health," the Productivity Commission reported. "People with mental illness are likely to be socially excluded, and people facing social exclusion for other reasons are likely to subsequently experience mental ill-health." Until we address this pattern of reviling difference, good-faith efforts at mental health reform will be – to a significant extent – more concerned with symptoms than with contributing causes and for that reason are likely to underperform or fail. This is for two reasons. First, the ways in which stigma is normalised in daily life will continue to exacerbate, and cause, poor mental health. Second, those who benefit from exclusionary norms are unlikely to fund evidence-based reforms.

When we focus on the social determinants of mental health and well-being, we get closer to addressing causes instead of symptoms. The idea is not new. In the Wurundjeri/Woiwurrung language, *Balit Durn Durn* means "strong brain, mind, intellect and sense of self." It was the title of the Victorian Aboriginal Controlled Community Health Organisation (VACCHO)'s report to the Royal Commission, and it is the header on the page setting out the Social and Emotional Wellbeing Wheel. This wheel has seven spokes: connection to one's body; connection to one's mind and emotions; connection to one's family and kinship; connection to Community; connection to Culture; connection to Country; and connection to spirit, spirituality and ancestors.

In Victoria, almost half of Aboriginal people have a relative who was stolen. Transgenerational trauma continues to affect Aboriginal people everywhere in Australia. The most recent data shows that 77 per cent of Aboriginal people aged eighteen to twenty-four who had experienced very high or high psychological distress had not seen a health professional. Indigenous health bodies have repeatedly explained that culturally safe clinical care – where the patient feels respected and empowered – would encourage better access. VACCHO's CEO, Jill Gallagher, has stated, "For too long, Aboriginal people have fallen through the cracks of a fragmented and culturally unsafe mental health system."

The Victorian Royal Commission recommended that a new Aboriginal Social and Emotional Wellbeing Centre be established, with recurrent funding for multidisciplinary teams inside Aboriginal health organisations. It also recommended funding a culturally appropriate service for children who require intensive support. Sheree Lowe, executive director of the new centre, believes that one of the positive things to come out of the Royal Commission is the adoption of the Aboriginal understanding of wellbeing, which is far broader than the medical model. "From our perspective," Lowe explains, "it's a holistic approach that's looking at more than just the clinical response to what people need. That's where the success is: to embed and understand those models and ways of doing things.

"If you look at the wheel – addressing one thing or taking one piece out of the puzzle, it will never completely work," she explains. "That's where, fundamentally, previous royal commissions have fallen down ... they've focused on one part, but not the whole.

"The history and impact for Aboriginal people in Australia is very real and very lived, and I think that's what people sometimes struggle with. That's why we hear comments in our national dialogues like, 'That happened in the past' and 'Why don't you just get over it?' My dad was born in 1954; he was born a non-citizen. He was a ward of the state by the age of fifteen. It wasn't until 1992 that Australia actually challenged and overturned the concept of terra nullius. If you think about that and you think about systemic racism and discrimination, the inclusion of Aboriginal people in the fabric of society is still very, very new.

"So, we've got to go through an un-learning process about what we've learnt through a Western education system that's left out critical factors around how colonisation occurred. That plays a big part in how we move forward, because if you don't have a sense of belonging and connection – and for us, a spiritual connection to land and seas – it has a massive contributing factor to mental health, wellbeing ... But for a lot of people, we're still fighting for access to those things that are an integral part of our healing and wellbeing.

"We often talk about if you get it right in this space ... everybody benefits from that. That's a core value for us; when we succeed, everybody succeeds. It's very rare for us that we live in the world of individualism, it's very collective-centred."

*

I am thinking what it means to remember. What would a literal re-membering look like? "If you boil the strange soup of contemporary right-wing ideology down to a sort of bouillon cube," Rebecca Solnit wrote in her 2016 essay, "The Ideology of Isolation," "you find the idea that things are not connected to other things, that people are not connected to other people, and that they are all better off unconnected. The core values are individual freedom and individual responsibility: yourself for yourself on your own."

Freud gestured towards this a century prior: "In the many different forms of obsessional neurosis in particular, forgetting is mostly restricted to dissolving thought-connections, failing to draw the right conclusions and isolating memories."

Opening the 2011 National Congress of Australia's First People, Lowitja O'Donoghue stated, "Since the 1967 referendum, Australia has been living a lie. It has patted itself on the back as a fair country, one that treats its citizens equally and, especially, protects the vulnerable." This gap between the ideal and the reality is where my mind returns as I read through the archives of the newspaper named for all of us:

> The largest four brand pillars of woke are gay, trans, gender, and race ... In reality, woke threatens to undermine the values of Western civilisation.

The leaders of the same-sex marriage campaign vociferously denied that the 2017 plebiscite was a threat to religious freedom. And yet that is what it has become.

When, in response to a question, Wallabies star Israel Folau posted on social media that he believed God's plan for gay people was hell 'unless they repent of their sins and turn to God,' he merely was expressing a view shared by many Christians, not to mention other religions ... That gay sex is a sin is a moral or religious view held by many Christians even though it is out of step with contemporary attitudes that accord equal rights to same-sex couples. But it is not hate speech or vilification.

Unfortunately, the Andrews government and senior police have equivocated at times about African gangs, as if the greater danger were an outbreak of mass racism among ordinary Victorians.

When someone is stigmatised, they are marked as different and lesser by the dominant culture, placed outside the circle of human concern. This happens under a cloak of normative invisibility– "just is-ness" – to those lucky and privileged enough not to be directly harmed by it. The result is sometimes termed "minority stress" and its consequences can be lethal. Carter Smith described this in a 2016 episode of Q+A discussing the concocted controversy over the Safe Schools program, which had been designed to combat prejudice by teaching students about the human realities of sexual and gender diversity. "I think the problem is politicians are using young, innocent, in-pain children as political bullets," Smith said. "This entire debate ... is still creating the idea that they are different, that they are wrong, that they are not accepted ... That is driving kids to hurt themselves, that is driving kids to kill themselves."

Statistically, the nine Australians who die every day by suicide are likely to have mental health issues and be male, Indigenous and/or LGBTIQ+.

As of April 2021, 53.2 per cent of queer people aged fourteen to twenty-one had considered suicide in the previous twelve months. Because "we are nodes on intricate systems, synapses snapping on a great collective brain," as Solnit eloquently phrased it, for each life lost to suicide the impacts are felt by up to 135 people, including family members, colleagues, friends, neighbours and first responders.

On the morning of census day in August 2021, I discussed youth suicide with Zed Tintor, deputy CEO of LGBTIQ+ Health Australia. "These are alarming statistics. We're seeing minority stress – the impacts of discrimination, internalised stigma, harassment, assault. It creates the conditions for poor mental health." Older people, Tintor explained, can at least draw on lived experiences of resilience in the face of prejudice, but young people are in the process of accumulating those experiences. "For a young person that's just entered this space, there's such high vulnerability and risk because the country is saying there's something wrong about me.

"Today is the census," they continued, "and our lives aren't included in it. The dominant structure is that of a heterosexual individual. For a young person seeing that – it's like, 'Where am I in this, why am I not included?' If this was a country that gives a fair go, we would see ourselves in the census … We've seen it with the Indigenous population, and with the different waves of immigration – how the Other has always been constructed as a danger to the structures that reinforce who we are as a culture."

*

There are other recent examples. Speaking on the Migration Amendment (Strengthening the Character Test) Bill 2019, federal ALP MP Julian Hill referred to "the Victorian Liberals' obsession before the state election with driving up community fear about South Sudanese gangs. The police actually said that in most cases there is no such gang; they don't exist. But that didn't stop the government … Of course, you would notice that most of that fear about South Sudanese gangs – 'We can't go out to dinner in

Melbourne' – stopped when the Liberals lost the state election. We don't hear much about that anymore, but we had twelve months of it."

Which brings me to September 2021, when Matthew Guy became Victoria's Liberal Opposition leader. Guy had stated in 2018 that Melbourne had "an issue with Sudanese gangs" and that the government was "allowing Melbourne to become the Johannesburg of the South Pacific."

"The consequences of the fear campaign, more like a racist campaign, were devastating and unrelating," wrote lawyer and human rights advocate Nyadol Nyuon in *The Age*. "Community legal centres reported a more than 50 per cent increase in racist attacks on African-Australians and other people of colour … A survey of 2500 people living across 150 suburbs in Melbourne by Associate Professor Rebecca Wickes of Monash University found that one in four people reported 'very low levels of warmth towards African people.'"

Nyuon made the point that although African-Australians were the targets of the race-based moral panic, they were not its only victims. "The divisive nature of that campaign sought to corrode and weaken the ties that bind us into a shared identity as Victorians." On becoming leader, Guy stated that he no longer thought Victoria had a problem with ethnic gang violence, partially because of the lockdowns. Should the Liberals win the 2022 state election, Guy would become premier, the person responsible for the reform of Victoria's mental health system.

Born in a refugee camp in Ethiopia after her family fled the Second Sudanese Civil War, Nyuon has spent much time and energy speaking out against racism in Australia, at considerable personal cost. Whenever she's done so, she's been the target of unrelenting online abuse. "Politically and in the media, we construe the conversation about racism as 'hurt feelings,'" she explains to me. "It's about 'being offended,' but what is lacking in the political and media narrative is the health consequences of racism and discrimination, including mental health." The 2014 Victorian Population Health Survey indicated that adults who frequently experience racism are almost five times more likely to have poor mental health.

Here is what Nyuon is seeing on the ground in South Sudanese and African communities: "I hear of at least two to three suicides of young people under the age of twenty-five in a month. Clearly there's a crisis. But it's a crisis in a minority community that is not really being responded to.

"Something like suicide, people say it's complicated, but I'm not sure whether we say that so we won't have to try to understand. I believe there is a significant contributing factor in the sense of isolation and being besieged, when you have media and politicians categorising people who look like you in a particular way. Those conversations don't just end as conversations; they have real impact. It does real damage. It begins to shift the very idea of how a kid thinks about themselves and what they are worthy of receiving.

"I think it comes from a perception of who really feels entitled to this country. There are people who really feel like Australia belongs to them, and other people are here in a hierarchical relationship and should know their place. Politically, it works to be able to generate anger from those who are losing that way of life. It's contributed to an environment where rage is clickbait. That makes it very hard for people to change their approach, because now there is almost an economic argument for engaging in it. Look at the kinds of people who are making the most money in the commentary space.

"During the 'African gangs crisis,' I could read an article and know whether they were talking about black or white kids, even if it didn't mention race. If it was Sudanese kids, the language that was used was the extreme language of fear. We are cultivated in a media environment and people can begin to understand that if they look at how the same media is covering climate change, or Covid-19 – the constant undermining of public health messages. That's also the damage that is done when they cover race. It's an exhausting way to live; it wears out your self-esteem and your mental health to carry other people's fear."

In *The Age*, Nyuon wrote: "I was reminded recently by Ajak Kwai, a prominent South Sudanese singer living in Melbourne, how raw everything still feels. She wrote that she wanted to disappear this time because she has no 'skin left to tolerate Matthew Guy.' She said: 'He left a big scare on us last time and now he is back and we [have] barely recovered from his wounds.'"

*

"All those creeks and crossings where Aboriginal people were massacred, buildings where children were institutionalised and abused, bits of Melbourne where Tracey Connelly and Jill Meagher were ambushed and killed . . . all waiting to haunt us into some new, essential knowledge about this world," Maria Tumarkin wrote in her 2015 essay "No Skin."

*

The day after a gallows and Trump flags are marched past the Victorian parliament in an anti-lockdown protest, I drive by that building: four or five protestors are camped out, laughing, on its stairs as the sun sets on the empty city. I am listening to clinical psychologist and Jungian psychoanalyst Donald Kalsched being interviewed about his 2020 essay "Wrestling with Our Angels: Inner & Outer Democracy in America Under the Shadow of Donald Trump."

He describes anxiety rising in the early Covid era, as bodies swiftly stacked up against a backdrop of racial inequality, economic inequality, the sixth extinction that is the climate crisis, and technological developments that have exponentially increased the ability to inflict mass violence, from drone warfare to domestic terrorism. Fear is exacerbated, Kalsched explains, anxiety too, and these are emotions we rarely allow ourselves to fully feel and around which our dissociative defences accumulate so that we don't have to.

"A great deal of what's going on in the culture right now under the title of 'fake news' is the denial of these realities that we really have to face as a people," he says. Not everyone can handle reality, "because they can't bear the feelings of grief that come up" and so – mostly unconsciously – they create an alternative one. This relationship to political or scientific fact mirrors an inward relationship to personal ones. We all repress feelings that conflict with our idealised images, but where someone's trauma background is particularly severe, those feelings might be so painful that they will be entirely dismembered, in a totalitarian act of repression.

What Kalsched calls a "democratic psychology," by contrast, is spacious enough to hold the good and bad aspects of ourselves and others. And just as it can sit with the distress of what has been endured personally, it is sufficiently robust to look unflinchingly at the surrounding world. Elements of both dissociative and democratic psychologies exist to a certain degree in everyone; however, the totalitarian system, with its polarised extremes of good and evil, tends to take over in times of stress or emotional overload – ejecting the painful aspects of reality from conscious experience. And, Kalsched maintains, the impulses that govern our interior lives also play out externally in our political patterns.

Denying social or scientific realities in our scrambling for safety means "we don't have to look at the vulnerability we're creating, the injuries we're creating, the unfairness of our society." We don't have to face the conflict that this, too, is us. All the time in psychotherapy, Kalsched explains, we're trying to get people to face all the parts of themselves they've marginalised and designated as bad: "one of the major defences is to vilify, shame and marginalise." Converting that frantically defensive energy into something more adapted to daily living requires, as electricity requires, a transformer. And that transformer, in Kalsched's analogy, is relationship.

"To be able to hold that conflict, the awareness that we, despite our good intentions, create evil in the world … It's not easy. It's the work of democracy and it's the work of psychology."

*

Photos of those gallows were on most news sites the day of the protest. Looking at that archaic instrument of death, instantly recognisable to the modern eye, I thought about the eternal return of those unaddressed patterns of the past. And how the site of Melbourne's first public execution is just around the corner from parliament.

There, in 1842, Tunnerminnerwait and Maulboyheenner, two Aboriginal men from Van Diemen's Land, became the first people to be hanged by the government in the District of Port Phillip. They had been convicted on circumstantial evidence for the murder of two whale-hunters. Intended to communicate a political message about resistance to colonisation, their hanging was "the biggest story of the day in the news-papers." Thousands watched as they died, slowly, at the end of ropes. "The gallows were in-expertly built ... and it seems, did not efficiently perform their function."

Both men were buried in unmarked graves in an unconsecrated section of the Old Melbourne Cemetery. When you stroll down the neat and bountiful rows of Queen Victoria Market, they are there still, just beneath your feet.

> Systems change, as a way of making real and equitable progress on
> critical social and environmental problems, requires exceptional
> attention to the detailed and often mundane work of noticing and
> acting on much that is implicit and invisible to many but is very
> much in the water.
>
> —John Kania, Mark Kramer and Peter Senge,
> *The Water of Systems Change*, 2018

At once bureaucratically blunt and opaque, "systems change" is a deceptively simple phrase. A first principle of systems change is that if we do not address the complex, interwoven root causes of social problems, the best-intentioned reform efforts "will only be mitigating the consequences of malfunctioning systems, or even providing inadvertent cover for their failure." Those surrounding conditions – the water we swim in, as Kania, Kramer and Senge term it, because such conditions are invisibly normative to many – include not just government policies but social conventions, market forces, power imbalances and knowledge gaps. Grappling with "this messy kaleidoscope of factors" is a different proposition to policy reform or changes in practices and resourcing. Change cannot only be structural; it must also be relational. As Katherine Whetton – the deputy secretary for mental health at the Victorian Department of Health – described it to me: "You can't plan your way through solving complex problems. Instead, these problems need to be solved over time through experimentation and iteration and shared learning."

So, if it's true, as Kania, Kramer and Senge write, that "transforming a system is really about transforming the relationships between people who make up the system," then there lies the probable explanation for our historical pattern of dead-ends. The same relational failures ("gaps") driving the crisis in the first place are also behind the failures to resolve it.

Seemingly radical in its recognition that restoring natural interconnectedness is the precondition for optimal human functioning, systems change is perfectly suited to remedying a problem that has, to a large degree, resulted from myriad forms of isolation, exclusion, erasure and estrangement. But while the philosophy is indeed at odds with most Western governance models, it is not new. That knowledge is Indigenous knowledge, crafted and applied by the oldest continuous culture on the planet.

Systems change is characterised by: curiosity, an emphasis on understanding of (and respect for) local contexts, power sharing over top-down leadership, self-reflection and personal accountability. Apart from being structural and relational, such change also needs to be mental. Those who hold power must do the interior work of identifying their own assumptions and prejudices. Likewise, an organisation's capacity to change is constrained by its own internal practices and norms.

In adopting a systems-change approach, the Victorian Royal Commission made a profound departure – other inquiries, like the Productivity Commission's, had framed arguments for reform largely according to the neoliberal model of a return on investment. Deep change cannot be superimposed on sociopolitical systems saturated with disparities and exclusionary norms. That is not, as the history of failure in the area shows us, how a paradigm shift works. It requires, instead, true metamorphosis: all structures shifting together, reinforcing one another, and overseen by conscious human actors who are modelling the changes they wish to see in the world.

*

Hippocrates and Galen used the word "crisis" to describe the turning point in a disease, the change pointing towards recovery or death. The history of Australia's mental health systems is one of sustained crisis. The Productivity Commission observed that while change was possible, "any notion that governments can dislodge deep-seated mental health issues within a term of government" should be dismissed. The Victorian Royal

Commission was similarly frank, saying that reform is a ten-year proposition requiring "unwavering commitment" from government and all partners. However, there will be three state elections before implementation is complete.

The commissioners' parting words emphasised that a new levy and dedicated capital investment fund was critical to lasting reform. The government subsequently introduced a bill imposing that tax – the mental health and wellbeing surcharge – on businesses with a national payroll greater than $10 million. Treasury framed the levy as less expensive than the direct annual cost to employers of poor mental health: $1.9 billion from lost productivity and workplace injuries. In his budget speech, Victorian treasurer Tim Pallas said the levy would affect less than 5 per cent of employers and framed it as payback for subsidies such as JobKeeper, mentioning that many big businesses profited despite the pandemic. Challenging the eleven crossbenchers to support the bill, Pallas stated that those familiar with the commission's work would know there was a crisis and that he would "simply appeal to their sense of fairness and reason."

"You don't help mental health by taxing people out of a job," said Michael O'Brien, then Opposition leader, who lobbied the crossbench to vote against the levy. Liberal MP David Davis called the levy "a huge, huge hit on Victoria's competitiveness": "I think it stigmatises mental health that they have put it as a special levy of this type." Liberal MP Gordon Rich-Phillips called it "a very substantial drag on the Victorian economy," and "a very substantial deterrent to job creation in this state." He continued: "We believe that mental health services are important. They are more important now than at any point in time because of the way in which this government has harmed the social fabric and has harmed the mental well-being of the Victorian community ... but they should be funded as the core base of government services, not through a tacked-on mental health and wellbeing levy."

Funding for mental health services is shared between federal, state and territory governments. The states typically pay over 60 per cent, the federal government 34 per cent, and third-party insurers 5.5 per cent. In 2018–19, the federal contribution worked out to $143 per person. The Victorian levy was criticised by the federal treasurer, Josh Frydenberg, whose 2021 allocation for national mental health – $2.3 billion – fell significantly below that of the Victorian commitment for a single state. The Victorian commitment also represented more than the total contribution made by every state and territory under the COAG National Action Plan on Mental Health 2006–2011 (around $3.5 billion). In doing so, Mental Health Australia observed, Victoria "recognised the scale of investment needed and set a bar for every jurisdiction."

I followed the levy debate, increasingly unable to reconcile the nature of the pushback with optimism about the imminence of transformative change. Succour came from an unlikely man. Despite "not [being] a fan of new taxes," Shooters, Fishers and Farmers Party MP Jeff Bourman supported the bill, as did seven more of the state's eleven crossbenchers. It passed. "If you're going to increase the services," Bourman said, "then it's got to come from somewhere." Australians tend to cast their vote on a conventional understanding of economic management and security. Bourman's rationale alluded not only to the longer view, but also to the incontrovertible human need at the heart of the matter.

In the taxonomy of politicians, there are those who consider their judges to be future generations and those more concerned with the immediate accrual of power. In its 2021 federal budget analysis, Mental Health Australia observed that a "longer-term vision for how mental health should work in, say, 2035 is perhaps the Budget's most glaring omission." In the debate over the Victorian levy, the speed with which a measure deemed "critical" by an independent public inquiry became politicised, and the specific nature and sources of that opposition, also bodes poorly for our future. It demonstrates magical thinking from politicians, who expect services and sectors to adhere to expert advice and empirical evidence, and to form collaborative connections, but are themselves unwilling to do this. It points to a perception by certain elected leaders that "the vulnerable" remain available for use as political bullets, to borrow Carter Smith's phrase. And that a swathe of the electorate will not only tolerate that behaviour but demand it.

The Victorian Chamber of Commerce and Industry said that while it welcomed the reforms, it was "disappointed that the government will hike up taxes for business and investors to fund core responsibilities." Gerry Harvey, owner of Harvey Norman, which doubled its profits during the pandemic, told *The Age* it was a "dreadful, horrible, stupid tax." Business Council of Australia chief executive Jennifer Westacott called the levy a "very dangerous precedent of fiscal repair which ultimately harms growth." "While we welcome mental health reform," she said, "which is much needed to deal with systemic issues and the devastating impact of a long and disproportionate lockdown, an approach that pits some Victorians against others by taxing jobs makes everyone a loser."

*

A new and sophisticated model of care-support that respects the human rights of people living with mental illness should be seen in the same light as a life-saving vaccine.

—Professor Kevin Bell, submission to the Royal Commission into Victoria's Mental Health System

The ex of a friend is against vaccination for ideological reasons, against mask-wearing. He is a father of young children, and not in particularly good health. Should he require hospitalisation for Covid-19, he will go to one of Australia's public hospitals, funded with taxes for the common good and which, as I write this, are rapidly filling with unvaccinated Covid patients relying on others to help them breathe. When he started posting memes, I went down the rabbit hole until I found this one: "If other people's health is now my responsibility, I assume it's legal for me to slap a McDonald's out of someone's hands and then chase them over an obstacle course?" It had so many likes I gave up trying to count them. Likes are a metric and, while they don't add up to much in the end, they do gesture towards the size of the substitute we have come to accept in the absence of authentic community.

At the end of last year, a GP described something they'd noticed across their small sample of patients who were adamant that the vaccine is harmful and part of a conspiracy. Most held strong religious or spiritual beliefs, a conviction that our present existence is just a prelude to a more glorious one. Also: limited education, low-paid work with little control over their destiny, and some degree of mental illness. Among the women, all had been subjected to abusive relationships and childhood trauma. Given that many with those characteristics don't hold such views, the doctor speculated that perhaps these factors were less important than time spent on the internet or watching Sky News, which remains the only mainstream Australian media outlet to have a YouTube video pulled for spreading vaccine misinformation. Perhaps, in the end, the only meaningful difference between "them" and "us" is whom we turn to for trustworthy information, and why. Who can blame them, the doctor said, for being short on trust in society at large, which has treated them so obscenely?

The sociologist Georg Simmel wrote that, in addition to the social life that is clearly visible, there exists between humans a multitude of minor relational forms and reciprocal effects which constitute the "unnamed or unknown tissue" that, in turn, creates society. In a previous Quarterly Essay, Margaret Simons wrote about the way a society isn't necessarily a community. Whereas societies are populations that "live in an ordered, rule-bound way, the relationships between them governed," a community recognises, and is bound by, common interest. This is a country where – before the pandemic – income inequality was above the OECD average. Housing is unaffordable. There is a gender pay gap. Low wage growth. Inequalities in the tax system, inadequacies in welfare payments, egregious racial disparities in our justice system. A significant overlap between conservative politics and private commercial interests. Insufficient investment in education, infrastructure and health. But while they seem increasingly vestigial these days, Australian democracy still has social-democratic reflexes.

From the relatively small turnout of the anti-lockdown protests, to the lack of unity in their aims and the American political language they employed, the lesson of Australia's pandemic response has not been "how easily we surrender our freedoms." The lesson is that a critical mass expects our governments to protect us when we are vulnerable and is willing to make sacrifices for the common good. The story is also that the government can mobilise, rapidly, to direct resources where they are needed. At one time, this was also the story told by our tax and housing and education and healthcare systems. The wheels started falling off decades ago, but the sentiment remains. In March 2019, also in a Quarterly Essay, Rebecca Huntley made the case, using granular research on social trends, that "[a] renewed form of social democracy is there for the making." "The majority of Australians would not only support it, they are demanding it," she wrote, "as seen in their attitudes to housing, the environment and democratic reform." One finding, however, that Huntley mentioned gnaws at me:

> When it comes to closing offshore detention centres ... there is division, with Essential showing Australians to be almost equally divided between keeping all asylum seekers on Nauru indefinitely, bringing only children and families to Australia, and closing the entire place and bringing all asylum seekers onshore for processing.

At its height, Australian social democracy not only existed alongside perpetual policing of monoculturalism – in short, a revulsion towards difference – it was perhaps, as Huntley pondered, the result of social cohesion reinforced by stories of common enemies. This sense of scarcity and precarity, and the malignant lack of empathetic imagination to which fear states give rise, has always been part of the colonial shadow. The point is not merely that we could find worthier grounds for unity amid our escalating mental health crisis. It's that if we want to fix what is broken, we will need to.

There is another lesson from the pandemic. In our conception of government, and our willingness to fund it, we are closer to the Nordic countries than to America. However, we're trending towards the latter with a new story of Australia. That story weaponises the language of individualism to advance inequality at increasingly dire cost. Its intended audience is the great Australian centre – already high valency for threat messaging – whom it seeks to radicalise because fear is a currency capable of conversion into clicks and votes and dividends. For that reason, the new story relies on a steady supply of Others as fresh targets on which to pin our own anxieties. In return for such threats identified (though not contained), the audience receives a sense of belonging, the synthetic safety that comes from shared righteous rage against a common enemy. And, as the decision to politicise the public health response to the pandemic has shown, the moral of this new story is freedom over equality, and one freedom above all – the freedom to be unbothered by others' needs, as Rebecca Solnit puts it.

However, as we continue to saw ourselves off our perch, mental health might be the great unifier that climate change and the pandemic aren't. A former director of America's National Institute of Mental Health, Thomas Insel, once said, "There's two kinds of families in America – there's families that are struggling with a mental illness and there's families that are not struggling with a mental illness yet." That applies to Australia, too. Which is why the far-reaching effects of our current mental health epidemic will ultimately reveal the new story of Australia for what it really is: the settlement's oldest story.

In a certain light, Australians are excellent at building community. In that light, we follow "the collectivist idea," as Geoffrey Blainey defined mateship in *The Tyranny of Distance*, "that men should be loyal to the men with whom they live and work." We love our kids, are good to our neighbours, and will stand in the dark to honour forebears who fought for future generations. However, consider again those piles of inquiries into our social ills and the light shifts to reveal other truths.

As shown by the present reality where ten women are hospitalised daily for injuries inflicted by a domestic partner, men are not reliably "loyal to those with whom they live." One police officer with three decades of experience told me that the mental health crisis presents most frequently and most distressingly as family violence – a call-out every five minutes – and that, as shocking as that figure sounds, it is a significant under-count. When we talk about family violence, we are talking about the mental health of those who experience it and those who perpetrate it. Our assumption that healthy families are the norm – that emotional literacy and regulation are universal default settings – is unjustified by the evidence, and continues to promote a culture of stigma and silence when it comes to family violence, child abuse and neglect. So it cannot truly be said yet that, collectively, we Australians are doing the right thing by those with whom we live. And when you look at what the electorate has done with decades' worth of knowledge about egregious institutional failures and their devastating human impacts, it cannot be said that we do the right thing by our neighbours, those with whom we work.

The main lie of the new story of Australia concerns time: it holds that things are inexorably getting better when, in fact, we are drowning. The problem is cardinal, by which I mean that *within* our micro-communities of family systems, dysfunction is too often the norm. And the problem is also ordinal – it lies in the vast emptiness *between* communities, those Other places which we regard, to the extent that we regard them at all, as burdens or threats. And in both failures we find traces of the old mentality – carceral, colonial – violently disavowing our intractable vulnerability and interdependency.

*

They say madness is doing the same thing and expecting a different outcome. In our ever-new impulse to right what is wrong through inquiry after inquiry, only to fail to hold governments to account when they ignore or cherrypick from the findings, it turns out it is us – the collective, the electorate, the body politic and the body psychic – that is unwell. Sitting with that discomfort, it's important not to move from "a world in which there are no shadows to one in which there is no light," as the art historian Arthur Danto described the shift in Goya's life marked by his 1794 painting *Yard with Lunatics*. Between unrealistic optimism and useless nihilism, there must be a third way.

Funding is vital. New, more and better services are vital. But unless we deal with the relational conditions that are creating and exacerbating mental illness in this country, demand will continue to overwhelm supply. If marginalisation, stigma and apathy are story-driven, so too are their antidotes. The stories shared by hundreds of traumatised people from all parts of society, who spoke before the Victorian Royal Commission about the excoriating human cost of the system we have run into the ground, are now publicly available. Those are the narratives that have the power to shift the mental models of a significant swathe of voters and taxpayers. They have the power to bring unlikely people into reflection, and relationship. But in a country whose attention to history has largely been limited to broadening the sphere of acceptable forgetting, the existence of these narratives is not enough. Because there is no systems change without relational change – and no relational change without personal change – perhaps our best hope lies in a critical mass of those who are privileged by the current economic and social model following the lead of those people with lived experience and making the radical choice to normalise their own vulnerabilities – not just by refusing to participate in the stigmatisation of mental illness, but by calling out Othering in all its pernicious forms. This would necessarily involve unwaveringly withholding support for politicians and corporations that fail to model meaningful change. As Katherine Whetton, the deputy secretary, said to me: while systems change requires a different mindset from government – "the reforms belong to all of us, and the government is only one part of the system driving and supporting change."

*

In July 2021, the federal government established the Royal Commission into Defence and Veteran Suicide. It is required to produce a final report by June 2023.

In January 2022, the assistant minister for mental health and suicide prevention, David Coleman – who was minister for immigration, citizenship, migrant services and multicultural affairs when an attempt was made to deport the Murugappan family, with their Australian-born child and toddler – commented on the opening of a new mental healthcare centre in Darwin: "Head to Health centres are designed to provide a welcoming, low stigma, 'no wrong door' entry point for adults to access mental health information, services and supports."

In December 2020, Prime Minister Scott Morrison – architect of the recent religious discrimination bill – announced plans to develop the country's first National Stigma and Discrimination Reduction Strategy for all Australians who live with mental illness. Public consultations will be held in 2022.

*

"We're building our mental health system from the ground up," Victorian premier Daniel Andrews said in March 2021. "That means a system that actually provides people the care they need early – before they reach the emergency department, and in too many cases, before it's too late."

Figure–ground perception in Gestalt psychology refers to our tendency to simplify the undifferentiated information of daily life into the main object (figure) and everything else (ground). A classic example is an image of a black vase on a white background. You'll first see only the vase or two people facing each other. This is our fallible sorting reflex at work – seeking false certainty over accuracy, reflexively grouping things by simple similarity or proximity, picking what's worth our energy and what we can ignore. It highlights that, while our perceptions are influenced by our biases and prejudices, we always have the power to look again. And that other possibilities exist between the interacting parts which comprise the whole.

What would happen if we became curious about the sources of our strangely ambivalent relationship to change? If we acknowledged the fact that our vulnerability is our greatest strength because it is the source of true connection? If it all no longer seemed contemptible to us, and we chose to make that the telos of the pandemic – the direction in which the pain of our many crises sent us, soaring? What life would open up to all of us on the other side?

SOURCES AND ACKNOWLEDGMENTS

I am grateful to everyone who shared their knowledge, experience and time with me for this essay. Quoted or not, your insights illuminated the terrain. Thank you.

1   "Australians today": J.P. Parkinson, "The Castle Hill lunatic asylum (1811–1826) and the origins of eclectic pragmatism in Australian psychiatry", *Australian and New Zealand Journal of Psychiatry*, 15(4), 1981: 319.

3   most of us had experienced it: *The Fifth National Mental Health and Suicide Prevention Plan*, Department of Health, Commonwealth of Australia, 2017.

3   "ever-presence of stigma and discrimination": Parliament of the Commonwealth of Australia, House of Representatives Select Committee on Mental Health and Suicide Prevention, *Mental Health and Suicide Prevention – Interim report*, 31 April 2021; Productivity Commission, *Inquiry Report into Mental Health*, Vol. 1, 2020: 21; Royal Commission into Victoria's Mental Health System, *Final Report: Summary and recommendations*, 2021: 16; Mental Health Australia, *Advice to the National Mental Health Commission: National Stigma and Discrimination Reduction Strategy*, November 2021; C. Groot et al., *Report on Findings from the Our Turn to Speak Survey: Understanding the impact of stigma and discrimination on people living with complex mental health issues*, 2020; SANE Australia, *National Stigma Report Card: Report on findings from the Our Turn to Speak survey*, 2020.

3   "deeply discredited", "We construct", etc.: Erving Goffman, *Stigma: Notes on the management of spoiled identity*, Penguin, 1963: 13, 15.

3   impacts are compounded: *The Fifth National Mental Health and Suicide Prevention Plan*, 39; SANE Australia, *A Life Without Stigma*, 2013; National Mental Health Commission, *Contributing Lives, Thriving Communities: Report of the National Review of Mental Health Programmes and Services*, 2014.

4   stigma can both cause and exacerbate poor mental health: Royal Commission into Victoria's Mental Health System, *Final Report*, Vol. 3, 2021: 531.

5   essentially the same throughout the nation: Productivity Commission, *Inquiry Report into Mental Health*, Vol. 1, 2020: 95.

5   numbers have likely risen during the pandemic: Melissa Cunningham, "'Absolutely flooded': Record numbers of women seek mental health help", *The Age*, 21 September 2020; Josh Nicholas, "Is there a mental health crisis? What Australian data reveals about impact of Covid lockdowns", *Guardian Australia*, 3 September 2021; Matt Wade, "Hidden costs: Lockdown toll on mental health

put at $13 billion", *The Sydney Morning Herald*, 24 January 2022; Melissa Cunningham, "Psychiatric beds closed as mental health crisis worsens under Omicron", *The Age*, 22 January 2022.

5   72 per cent of secondary teachers: Royal Commission into Victoria's Mental Health System, *Final Report*, Vol. 2, 2021: 83.

5   a mental health call-out about every twelve minutes: Victoria Police, *Submission to the Royal Commission into Victoria's Mental Health System*, 5 July 2019: 3.

5   approximately 3189 people presented: Austin Health, *Submission to the Royal Commission into Victoria's Mental Health System*, 8 July 2019: 8.

5   3.3 million missing hours: Royal Commission into Victoria's Mental Health System, *Fact Sheet: Community-based mental health and wellbeing services*.

5   most Australians do not seek help: Nicholas, "Is there a mental health crisis?"; SANE Australia, *Fact vs Myth: Treatment & recovery*, 2016; Productivity Commission, *Inquiry Report into Mental Health*, Vol. 3, Australian Government, 2020: 1262.

7   "For too long": Royal Commission into Victoria's Mental Health System, *Interim Report*, 2019: 12.

7   "A human relationship": Carl Jung, *Civilisation in Transition*, Princeton University Press, 1964, p. 301.

8   "centred on transformational reform": Victorian Government, "Announcement: Royal Commission into Mental Health Speech", 24 October 2018.

8   "to rebalance": Royal Commission into Victoria's Mental Health System, *Final Report, Summary and recommendations*, 2021: 20.

8   "mental health is shaped": Royal Commission into Victoria's Mental Health System, *Final Report*, Vol. 1: 150.

8–9   "Inquiries are not new in mental health": Ian Hickie and Sebastian Rosenberg, *The Conversation*, 30 October 2018.

9   no fewer than 14: Productivity Commission, *Inquiry Report into Mental Health*, Vol 2: 103, fn. 4.

9   "business as usual": Jennifer Doggett, "Do it better or do it differently?", *Inside Story*, 10 December 2017.

9   "Despite numerous past inquiries": Productivity Commission, *Productivity Commission Inquiry Report into Mental Health*, 2(95), 2020: 103, fn. 4.

9   over 500 Aboriginal deaths in custody: Lorena Allam, "'Beyond heartbreaking': 500 Indigenous deaths in custody since royal commission", *Guardian Australia*, 6 December 2021.

10   "there are few, if any": Mental Health Australia, *Federal Budget Analysis*, 28 May 2021.

10   "that the patient": Sigmund Freud, "Remembering, repeating and working-through" in *Further Recommendations on the Technique of Psychoanalysis*, 1914.

10   "sickness unprevented for all our diligence": John Donne, *Devotions upon Emergent Occasions*, 1627.

11   one of the most marginalised sections: See, for example, David Andrew Roberts, "The 'Knotted Hands that Set Us High': Labour history and the study of convict Australia", *Labour History*, 100, 2011: 33; D. Meredith and D. Oxley, "Contracting convicts: The convict labour market in Van Diemen's Land 1840–1857", *Australian Economic History Review*, 45, 2005.

11   "a bare subsistence level": James Dunk, *Bedlam at Botany Bay*, NewSouth Books, 2019, p. 5, citing Lois Davey, Margaret Macpherson and F.W. Clements, *The Hungry Years: 1788–1792*, MUP, 1947, pp. 9, 15.

11   "bloody sight of corpses", "even if they avoided", "where discipline, security and industry", "Little of the colony's madness": Dunk, *Bedlam at Botany Bay*, pp. 2–3, 17–18.

12   "The stories of 'the killing times'": Lorena Allam and Nick Evershed, "The killing times: The massacres of Aboriginal people Australia must confront", *Guardian Australia*, 4 March 2019.

13   "According to traditional gender norms", etc.: Pauline Grosjean, "History repeating: Toxic masculinity and Australia's convict past", *The Conversation*, 29 March 2021.

14   higher than that of the United Kingdom, New Zealand and Canada: Australia has a suicide rate of 12.5 per 100,000; Canada's is (like that of Norway, Iceland and the Netherlands) 11.8; New Zealand's is 11; the United Kingdom's is 7.9.

14   "That was before": Doggett, "Do it better or do it differently?"

14   1.9 per cent of deaths: Australian Bureau of Statistics, *Deaths, Australia*, ABS, 29 September 2021; Australian Bureau of Statistics, *Causes of Death, Australia*, ABS, 29 September 2021.

14   suicide was the leading cause of death among Australian children and adolescents: Australian Institute of Health and Welfare, *Suicide and intentional self-harm*, AIHW, 23 July 2020.

14   mental ill-health was present in around 90 per cent of young people who died by suicide: Orygen, *Raising the Bar for Youth Suicide Prevention*, 2016.

14   double that of the non-Indigenous population: AIHW, *Deaths by suicide amongst Indigenous Australians*, 18 October 2021.

14   "exceptionally high": K. Hedrick et al., "Self-harm among asylum seekers in Australian onshore immigration detention: How incidence rates vary by held detention type", *BMC Public Health*, 2020: 592.

16   this diagnosis: See, for example, Andrew M. Chanen, "Bigotry and borderline personality disorder", *Australasian Psychiatry*, 29(6) (2021): 579.

16   approximately 6 per cent: F.S. Brin et al., "Personality disorder: A mental health priority area", *Australia & New Zealand Journal of Psychiatry*, 51(9) (2017): 872.

17   In the frosty language: F.S. Brin et al., "Personality disorder".

17   "In view of the substantially increased stress levels": Martin Bohus et al., "Borderline personality disorder", *The Lancet*, 398, 2021: 1528.

18   "The diagnosis of BPD has few friends": Andrew M. Chanen, "Bigotry and borderline personality disorder", *Australasian Psychiatry*, 29(6), 2021: 579.

19   For Australians living with schizophrenia: SANE Australia, *Media release: Decrease in suicide rates is not a time for celebration*, 20 August 2020.

19   174 young people in custody: Youth Parole Board: *Annual Report 2018–19*, State of Victoria Department of Justice and Community Safety, September 2019.

22   A quarter of the state's homeless population: Jewel Topsfield, "'Terrifying, cold and a lot of loud noises': Homeless young people falling through safety net", *The Age*, 4 August 2021.

22   build over 12,000 homes: Jewel Topsfield and Royce Millar, "'This will change lives': $5.2 billion social-housing construction blitz", *The Age*, 15 November 2020.

25   "outside conventional education": Dr Marnee Shay, quoted in the University of Queensland, "A flexible approach to learning: Can flexi schools close the gap for Indigenous learners?", https://stories.uq.edu.au/research/2020/a-flexible-approach-to-learning/index.html, accessed 20 February 2022.

26   "My supervisor said": *This Jungian Life*, Episode 74, "Borderline Personality Disorder", 29 August 2019.

27   "we have almost an inherent blindness to it": Hayley Foster quoted in Wendy Tuohy, "Nearly 3 million Australians have survived sexual violence", *The Sydney Morning Herald*, 24 August 2021.

28   one in six women and one in nine men: AIHW, *Australia's children*, 3 April 2020.

28   "gaps in non-acute services in communities lead to avoidable hospital admissions": Productivity Commission, *Inquiry Report into Mental Health*, Vol 1, p. 36.

28   risen by about 70 per cent: Productivity Commission, *Inquiry Report into Mental Health*, Vol. 1, p. 28.

29   "provide a range of therapeutic interventions and programs": Department of Health, *Acute Inpatient Services*, 29 May 2015.

30   "supreme end of man's endeavour": "Introduction" to Cicero, *De Finibus*, Harvard University Press, 1931.

30   "I find myself": *This Jungian Life*, "Borderline Personality Disorder".

31   raped in the community: Frequency of sexual assault of children in residential care: Victorian Ombudsman, *Investigation into Complaints about Assaults of Five Children Living in Child Protection Residential Care Units*, 2020.

32   Children who witness family violence in the household are more likely to re-engage with the justice system in the future: Crime Statistics Agency, *Data Snapshot: Child witnesses of family violence: An examination of Victoria Police family violence data*, February 2021.

32   "serious lack": Rachel Dexter, "'This work is not done': Children still dying amid family violence", *The Age*, 30 March 2021.

33   sixty-five children in Victoria who were known to child protection authorities died: Dexter, "'This work is not done'".

33   only 20 per cent of children: Productivity Commission, *Inquiry Report into Mental Health*, Vol. 2: 250.

35   "stunning decision": Frances Vinall, "Psychologist would 'rather have schizophrenia' than this severe disorder", *The Australian*, 25 August 2020.

35   "By definition": Goffman, *Stigma*.

35   "charge of stigmatization": Susan Sontag, *Illness as Metaphor & Aids and Its Metaphors*, Penguin, 1981, p. 101.

35   BPD, uniquely, did not count for the purposes of exoneration or mitigation: The situation in other jurisdictions of Australia varies. Sometimes it is accepted, other times not. Post-O'Neill, some of the other states (for example, Tasmamia) accepted the Victorian approach and excluded it, and some (for example, New South Wales) seemed a little more generous without properly addressing the issue at the level of principle.

35   Mystery persists: Bohus et al., "Borderline personality disorder".

36   neurobiological hypotheses: J.A. Coan and D.A. Sbarra, "Social baseline theory: The social regulation of risk and effort", *Current Opinions in Psychology*, 1, 2015: 87; Catherine Winsper, "The aetiology of borderline personality disorder (BPD): Contemporary theories and putative mechanisms", *Current Opinion in Psychology*, 21, 2018: 105.

37   neurobiologists continue to investigate: Winsper, "The aetiology of borderline personality disorder (BPD)"; Carla Sharp et al., "The structure of personality pathology: Both General ('g') and Specific ('s') Factors?", *Journal of Abnormal Psychology*, 124(2), 2015: 387; Bohus et al., "Borderline personality disorder".

39   "a community that would not help": *Attorney-General v David* [1992] VicRp 53, per Hedigan J. In reviewing David's continued detention, the court made reference to his "Blueprint for Urban Warfare," detailing, among other things, "the poisoning of city water supplies, the bombing of Flinders Street Station and the MCG on major sporting events, the bombing of major bridges and Zionist centres, the execution of the Premier and Prime Minister, the desire to be Australia's worst civilian mass murderer, the bombing of St. Vincent's Hospital, Melbourne, indiscriminate gunfire into crowded public places, the pouring of flammable liquids over crowds from high vantage points, the release of toxic poisons into public swimming pools, injection of AIDS contamination into milk cartons, the release of foot and mouth disease, bombing of crowded churches, universities, airports, major shopping retail outlets, Luna Park, TV studios, the indiscriminate shooting into crowds at Carols by Candlelight, freeways, bombing of airport facilities, the total devastation of the prison's office and the recreation of the Hoddle Street, Queen Street, Russell Street and Walsh Street massacres, with high death tolls in the same locations and on the same dates." The court also referred to threats he made to his doctors. "In violent and angry language he claimed that he was "insanely and violently angry" with them for abandoning him," Justice Hedigan noted. "He accused them, falsely as I judge, for failing to prepare him for the outside world and wanting to bury him under the carpet and forget him ... He said that he was terrified of going outside the walls but soon he would be forced outside ... He said that he could not survive, and that all he could do was to sacrifice himself in a very public and violent way. He ... reiterated how he was filled with rage and violent, blinding hatred against a community that would not help him to become part of it."

40   proportion of offenders with personality disorders could be around 40 per cent: Tony Butler et al., "Mental disorders in Australian prisoners: A comparison with a community sample', *Australia New Zealand Journal of Psychiatry*, 40(3), 2006: 272.

40   The lack of a more nuanced approach: Jaimie Walvisch, Andrew Carroll and Tim Marsh, "Sentencing and mental disorder: The evolution of the Verdins principles, strategic interdisciplinary advocacy and evidence-based reform", *Psychiatry, Psychology and Law*, 2021: 1.

52   the more information they have, the less punitive they are: Kate Warner et al., "Public judgement on sentencing: Final results from the Tasmanian Jury Sentencing Study", *Trends & Issues in Crime and Criminal Justice*, 407, Australian Institute of Criminology, 2011.

56   "must have been designed": Pauline Conolly, "Yarra Bend Asylum Cemetery," https://paulineconolly.com/2017/yarra-bend-cemetery.

60–1   "Specifically, the devastating effect of incarceration": Office of the Public Advocate, *Submission – Cultural review of the adult custodial corrections system*, 31 December 2021.

63   "a gentle eminence": John Conolly, *The Construction and Government of Lunatic Asylums and Hospitals for the Insane*, Dawsons, 1847.

66   an Indigenous man with fetal alcohol syndrome: Office of the Public Advocate, "The Illusion of 'Choice and Control': The difficulties for people with complex and challenging support needs to obtain supports under the NDIS", 2018; Adam Cooper, "Unconvinced, Indigenous, disabled man is free after 543 days in jail", *The Age*, 18 June 2018. Ruth McCausland and Eileen Baldry, "'I feel like I failed him by ringing the police': Criminalising disability in Australia", *Punishment & Society*, 19(3), 2017: 290.

66   "systematically criminalised": McCausland and Baldry, "'I feel like I failed him by ringing the police": Criminalising disability in Australia", *Punishment & Society*, 19(3), 2017: 290.

69   "enormous capacity": The Australian Women's Register, "Frost, Phyllis Irene (1917–2004)"

70   "bleak": Victorian Ombudsman, *Implementing OPCAT in Victoria: Report and inspection of the Dame Phyllis Frost Centre*, 2017: 52.

77   people with disability in Australia are at a significantly greater risk of experiencing physical and sexual violence: Centre of Research Excellence in Disability and Health, *Violence Against People with Disability in Australia*, 2017.

77   women with an intellectual or psychological disability: ABS, *Disability and Violence – In Focus: Crime and Justice Statistics*, 13 April 2021.

78   "About 4000", "In the community" Jewel Topsfield and Royce Millar, "How Denise Morgan escaped Albert Park's house of horrors", *The Age*, 27 September 2021.

78   "deplorable": Rebecca Opie, "SA coroner calls for national register of aggressive incidents at aged care homes", *ABC News*, 28 September 2018.

78   "Someone who is perennially": Susan Sontag, *Regarding the Pain of Others*, Farrar, Straus and Giroux, 2003.

79   "not only to address": Department of Human Services, *Because Mental Health Matters: Victorian Mental Health Reform Strategy 2009–2019*, 2009, 29; Royal Commission into Victoria's Mental Health System, *Final Report: Summary and recommendations*, Vol. 1, 2021: 53.

79   "The system is achieving": *Witness Statement of Associate Professor Simon Stafrace*, 7 July 2019, paras 146 and 148 cited in Royal Commission into Victoria's Mental Health System, *Final Report*, Vol. 1, 2021: 53.

79–80 "A sample": P. Wells, "The need for mental health services for adolescents in the Hunter Region", *Australian & New Zealand Journal of Psychiatry*, 14(4), 1981: 355.

80   four-month waitlist: Adrian Plaskett, "It's rare to be able to tell the truth – here's what's wrong with Australia's mental health system", *Guardian Australia*, 26 April 2021.

81   more than half: Domain Rental Report, September 2021; ABS, *Australian National Accounts: National Income, Expenditure and Product*, 1 December 2021.

86 The Royal Commission found: Royal Commission into Victoria's Mental Health System, *Fact Sheet: Community-based mental health and wellbeing services.*

91 "For Indigenous peoples": Pat Dugeon et al., Solutions that Work: What the evidence and our people tell us – Aboriginal and Torres Strait Islander Suicide Prevention Evaluation Project report, 2016.

91 at a macro level: Matthew Clair, "Stigma" in *Core Concepts in Sociology*, John Wiley & Sons, 2018.

91 "that the normal": Rosemarie Garland-Thomson, "Reflections on the Fiftieth Anniversary of Erving Goffman's *Stigma*", *Disability Studies Quarterly*, 34(1), 2014.

92 "Social exclusion": Productivity Commission, *Productivity Commission Inquiry Report into Mental Health*, Vol. 1, 2020: 15.

92 *Balit Durn Durn*: VACCHO, *Balit Durn Durn: Strong brain, mind, intellect and sense of self*, Report to the Royal Commission into Victoria's Mental Health System, VACCHO August 2020.

92–3 Indigenous health bodies: Tracy Westerman, "Engaging Australian Aboriginal youth in mental health services", *Australian Psychologist*, 45, 2010: 212; Shirley McGough, Dianne Wynaden and Michael Wright, "Experience of providing cultural safety in mental health to Aboriginal patients: A grounded theory study", *International Journal of Mental Health Nursing*, 27, 2018: 204.

94 "If you boil": Rebecca Solnit, "The ideology of isolation", *Harper's Magazine*, July 2016.

94 "In the many different forms": Sigmund Freud, "Remembering, repeating and working-through".

94 "the largest four brand pillars"; Sean Masters, "Woke is a genius brand, and a threat to our way of life", *The Australian*, 21 May 2021.

94 "The leaders of the same-sex marriage campaign": Nick Cater, "Left anoints itself as the only true religion", *The Australian*, 7 December 2020.

95 "When, in response to a question": Editorial, "Tackling belief and free speech", *The Australian*, 11 April 2018.

95 "Unfortunately, the Andrews government": Editorial, "Melbourne's African gangs", *The Australian*, 30 December 2018.

95 "I think the problem": *Q+A*, ABC TV, 21 March 2016.

95 "we are nodes": Solnit, "The ideology of isolation".

96–8 "The consequences" etc.: Nyadol Nyuon, "'Brutal, dehumanising': African community remembers Liberal campaign", *The Age*, 10 September 2021.

97 adults who frequently: Royal Commission into Victoria's Mental Health System, *Final Report*, Vol. 3, 2021: 215.

98–9 "All those creeks and crossings": Maria Tumarkin, "No skin", 2 September 2015.

100 Intended to communicate: Clare Land, *Tunnerminnerwait and Maulboyheenner: The Involvement of Aboriginal People from Tasmania in Key Events of Early Melbourne*, City of Melbourne, 2014.

100–1 "biggest story of the day": Leonie Stevens, "The phenomenal coolness of Tunnerminnerwait", *Victorian Historical Journal*, 8(1), 2010: 18–40; Land, *Tunnerminnerwait and Maulboyheenner*.

101 "The gallows were": Land, *Tunnerminnerwait and Maulboyheenner*.

102 "will only be mitigating": Rob Abercrombie, "A shock to the system", NPC blog 23 June 2015.

103 "an organisation's capacity to change": John Kania, Mark Kramer and Peter Senge, *The Water of Systems Change*, FSG, 2018, p. 5.

104 funding for mental health services is shared: Amanda Biggs and Lauren Cook, *Health in Australia: A quick guide*, Parliamentary Library Research Paper Series, 2018–19, August 2018.

104–5 The states typically pay: AIHW, *Mental health services in Australia: Expenditure on mental health-related services*, updated 1 February 2022.

105 $143 per person: Cook, *Mental Health in Australia*.

105 "recognised the scale" and "longer-term vision": Mental Health Australia, *Federal Budget Analysis*, May 2021.

105 "If you're going": "Victoria's mental health levy is set to become law after passing state's upper house", *SBS News*, 9 June 2021.

106 "disappointed that": Calla Wahlquist, "From 'horrible and dreadful' to 'true reform at last': Reactions to Victoria's mental health levy", *Guardian Australia*, 21 May 2021.

106 "dreadful, horrible": Cara Waters, "'A kick in the guts': Business owners rail against mental health levy", *The Age*, 20 May 2021.

106 "very dangerous precedent" and "While we welcome": Calla Wahlquist, "From 'horrible and dreadful' to 'true reform at last'.

107 "live in an ordered, rule-bound way,": Margaret Simons, *Cry Me a River: The tragedy of the Murray–Darling River*, Quarterly Essay 77, March 2020.

108 can mobilise, rapidly: The Treasury, Australian Government, Economic Response to Covid-19 ("The 2021–22 Budget committed an additional $41 billion in direct economic support, bringing total support since the beginning of the pandemic to $291 billion as of May 2021.")

108 "[a] renewed form of social democracy is there for the making": Rebecca Huntley, *Australia Fair: Listening to the nation*, Quarterly Essay 73, March 2019.

109 "that men should be loyal": Geoffrey Blainey, *The Tyranny of Distance: How distance shaped Australia's History*, Sun Books, 1966, p. 171.

110   "loyal to those with whom": Our Watch, *Quick facts*, www.ourwatch.org.au/
       quick-facts accessed 20 February 2022.
109   "the collectivist idea": Blainey, *The Tyranny of Distance*.
110   significant under-count: Tuohy, "Nearly 3 million Australians".
111   "a world in which there are no shadows": Arthur Danto, "Shock of the Old:
       Arthur C. Danto on three Goya biographies", *Artforum International*, March 2004.

Hannah Ryan & Gina Rushton

What comes after the story? #MeToo relies on the idea that storytelling is revolutionary, but the ability of the movement to deliver accountability has always hinged on what follows the accounts of harassment that it demands people divulge.

Adrienne Rich wrote that when a woman tells the truth, she creates "the possibility for more truth around her." The victories of the movement have been won in these truthful spaces excavated by each disclosure. It is through stories that we unearth not just sexual harassment and violence, but the lengths to which institutions go in minimising, justifying, excusing, denying and hiding it.

Jess Hill records how the #MeToo movement has always derived power from storytelling – a chorus of survivors speaking together to testify that this harm is common, but unacceptable. The essay maps the courage and tenacity of the survivors who have spoken up, spoken out and spoken back over the past five years.

Telling these stories has not been easy, in part because of our stifling defamation laws and the legal caution exacerbated by the recklessness of the *Daily Telegraph*'s Geoffrey Rush story. But some survivors, and the frontline service providers and advocates who fight for them, were also let down by the way the #MeToo movement initially unfolded here – as covered by our reporting, which Hill references in her essay. Our investigation documented the formation of NOW Australia, the local version of Time's Up, co-founded by Tracey Spicer, who became the face of the nation's #MeToo movement in October 2017 when she asked people to bring her their stories following the Harvey Weinstein allegations.

By September 2019, Spicer claimed she had more than 2500 disclosures, and we found some had not been responded to. Amelia, a woman who disclosed to Spicer for the first time her harassment by a media figure, told us she gave up expecting a reply and assumed what happened to her wasn't "violent" enough to warrant one.

"Women sending information will be offered counselling and any support they need," Spicer told a newspaper, later publicly claiming to have connected "every person who has disclosed to me" to lawyers or counsellors.

The danger of a single person taking carriage of so many disclosures was further exposed in our subsequent series with Nina Funnell and news.com.au, in which we revealed the violation of survivors' privacy in a documentary, starring Spicer, about the #MeToo movement in Australia. An early version, which included the real names, faces and personal stories of rape and domestic violence victims, was circulated to media without the survivors' knowledge or consent. They had no knowledge their confidential disclosures had been shared with a film crew, and one woman told Funnell: "I didn't consent and she hasn't told me she would use my information in this way."

This is an egregious example, but how many times have we watched survivors lose control of their own stories as they are co-opted by media or political interests? After actor Eryn Jean Norvill's private complaint became tabloid fodder and she was dragged through a defamation trial, she stood outside the courtroom and said: "As you all know, I never wanted these issues to be dealt with by a court." When Catherine Marriott's report of sexual misconduct by Barnaby Joyce was leaked to the press, she said all her control had been "taken away." When journalist Ashleigh Raper's allegations of sexual harassment by the former NSW Labor leader were aired under parliamentary privilege by a political rival, she said it had happened without her "involvement or consent."

Does this loss of autonomy and control not reinscribe the same dynamic of disregarding someone's consent? As Hill acknowledges, people are denied the ability to tell their stories on their own terms, and even when they can, they risk public scrutiny and legal retaliation. If the movement is going to continue to gain muscle and momentum from survivors presenting their trauma so as to repeatedly prove the endemic nature of harassment and violence, we need to get better at protecting them. It is from storytelling that the movement has always drawn its power and it is the storytelling that exposes survivors to further harm. A public disclosure cannot be the template for driving reform when it comes to sexual harm. What comes after the story?

Last year's Australian of the Year, Grace Tame, found a trauma-informed and empathetic journalist in Funnell and, with other survivors, they campaigned to overturn gag laws preventing survivors from publicly identifying themselves. This is arguably an example of a story delivering material change – but even here, a young survivor of child sexual abuse has had to repeatedly retell her story at great personal cost. As Tame tells Hill, she was recently in the ER and lives "constantly on the precipice of a shame state from the retraumatisation." She helped overturn laws so that survivors could tell their story, not to insist they should.

Hill ends her essay by asking whether we are "winning" this war. We can take stock in many ways: In 2022, is a woman who tells her story of abuse or harassment in a different position than those who did so in 2017? Is she more likely to be heard and believed? Is justice more within her reach? Does she have greater access to help and healing? Does this access still differ based on her race, sexuality, disability or socioeconomic status? Most importantly, is a woman any less likely to have such a story? In other words, is sexual abuse and harassment any less prevalent because of #MeToo? (The statistics would say no.)

Glowing media coverage of NOW promised a triage service that would direct survivors to legal support, counselling and journalists as tensions ran high between Spicer and board members over what they could realistically achieve. The organisation folded in 2020 and became a cautionary tale – not only in how a well-intentioned group lacking infrastructure and experience can collapse under the weight of its own expectations, but also in the effects of over-promising and under-delivering to survivors of sexual violence. The irony was that if NOW had come through, it might have connected the hashtag to "the work," as Tarana Burke requested and Hill summarised as "grassroots activism, actual expertise in dealing with sexual violence, and the mission of structural change." If it had been better funded, if it had addressed the genuine concerns about diversity and the needs of women outside the arts, if it had spent time consulting with the sector about how to support people after their disclosures, if it had garnered political will and funding to deliver that, it might have been able to offer something material to survivors.

Success should continue to be measured by what we offer those who have stories to tell – whether or not they want to tell them. Instead of leaning towards the ears of survivors and saying, as our prime minister did to Tame, "Well, gee, I bet it felt good to get that out," we might have listened closer that day when she said, and as many survivors express, "Lived experience informs structural and social change."

Hannah Ryan & Gina Rushton

Amber Schultz

"Turning incuriosity into performance art": this is the line that stood out to me from Jess Hill's *The Reckoning*. Hill was referring to how, when Scott Morrison received an unsigned police statement alleging that, as a teenager, his right-hand man, Christian Porter, had raped a young girl named Kate, he hadn't even bothered to look at it. (Porter denies the allegation.)

The phrase perfectly encapsulates why the #MeToo movement was so powerful. Every woman knows a woman who has experienced sexual violence, but few men claim to know perpetrators. Why? Sheer incuriosity and utter disbelief that their friend, their mate, their bro could commit something so vile.

Or perhaps, when it came to Morrison's ministry and those on the other side of the political spectrum, it was something darker: if one could fall, so too could others. The Big Swinging Dicks club had to be protected at all costs.

When I first saw Alyssa Milano's #MeToo tweet trending, I was highly sceptical. Surely everyone knew harassment was rife? Society's tolerance for it was incredibly high. But women sharing examples and tales of abuse struck a chord. Yes, the prevalence of harassment was well known among women – but not, as I had assumed, among men. Or maybe I assumed men knew but didn't care, which, again as Hill notes, wasn't true.

As more and more stories were shared, memories – frustrating and frequent examples of harassment and abuse, which we had either pushed to the dark recesses of our brains or convinced ourselves we'd somehow caused – emerged and were reframed as what they really were.

Each shared individual experience was a small piece of the puzzle that, when joined together, helped us see the all-encompassing and pervasive culture of power, sexism and discrimination.

Such documentation is the heart of the #MeToo movement, as founder Tarana Burke intended it. Not necessarily finger-pointing – though, as Hill observes, this has added fire to the movement – but documenting abuse and harassment, however big and however small.

But once the puzzle was laid bare, not everyone wanted to look at it – especially those in parliament. So, when Brittany Higgins woke up half-naked on a couch in Parliament House, the room was deep-cleaned and the incident swept under the rug. When thousands of women and allies rallied outside parliament demanding action on sexual violence, they were ignored and told to be grateful they hadn't been shot. When the rape allegation against Porter emerged, he was an "innocent man" in Morrison's eyes.

See no evil, hear no evil, speak no evil.

I truly believe Morrison thought all the issues that came to light across 2020 might just ebb away, like many of his other public gaffes. But Australia had reached a tipping point. The silence simply made us louder, angrier and more driven. The Morrison government faced a dilemma: by the time Morrison began to address women's anger, he had already lost control of the narrative.

The progression in how Morrison talks about sexual violence has been morbidly fascinating to watch. If it weren't so rage-inducing, it would be comic – how frequently he got things wrong, squirmed as he tried to respond to difficult questions with spin to make himself look good, and made remarks he thought were clever but that showed a fundamental misunderstanding of the issue.

His rhetoric has improved: no longer does he evoke fatherhood or sympathy for "Jenny and the girls," refusing to acknowledge women as autonomous beings outside of their relationship to men. Now he tells women he gets it, he understands: sexual violence is bad.

But Morrison missed the starting gun – something palpably painful for him. He always tries to stay ahead of the narrative. When Morrison fields journalists' questions, he is in control. He'll avoid hosting press conferences when prickly issues emerge, telling journalists there'll be "another time" for answering their questions. There never is.

This is why, when sex discrimination commissioner Kate Jenkins' *Set the Standard* report dropped, Morrison hosted a press conference fifteen minutes after it was published and two hours before Jenkins hosted her own conference. He took the opportunity to pat himself on the back, stressing how much he had learnt from his one-hour training on gendered violence. He didn't specify what had been so revelatory.

When former NSW premier Gladys Berejiklian resigned, he quickly primed her for a federal seat, proudly announcing she had "a lot more to contribute" to politics. He was trying to use her as a political pawn, shoehorning her into a position she didn't want. When he faced criticism, he played the victim.

"People can't have it both ways," he said. "They can't say, why aren't you getting more women into parliament, and when I try and get women into parliament, and when it doesn't happen, they attack me."

Or like when former Liberal MP Julia Banks decided she would step down, unable to tolerate Morrison and his "menacing controlling wallpaper" presence. She agreed to not speak to the media for twenty-four hours, thinking she was being collegial – only to find out Morrison's office had started to background journalists about her, painting her as everything from a "weak petal" to a "bully."

But when it comes to the #MeToo movement, Morrison has lost control of the narrative. He tries to stay ahead of it, appointing himself as the keynote speaker of the Women's Safety Summit and dragging the Minister for Women, Linda Reynolds – who rarely speaks for more than a few minutes – to every press conference relating to gender.

But his attempts are too little, too late.

This is why Hill's essay is so powerful. It lays down the narrative, without spin but with deep analysis, adding perspective to two years of anger and inaction.

It displays the entire puzzle in a clear light for all to see.

Amber Schultz

Malcolm Knox

Jess Hill's Quarterly Essay is, like all her work, a powerful example of how anger can be artfully harnessed to thorough, evidence-based, utterly convincing argument. Even if you already accepted the sentiment and thought you knew the facts, Hill's essay renews the energy for change.

In her final pages, she raises the most urgent questions for men who hold themselves innocent of harassing, abusing, raping, objectifying and coercing: men who are also angry, without having been direct victims themselves, yet tentative about entering the debate and who do not quite know how to help. Hill asks: "What right do men have to talk about #MeToo? Do we as women really want them in this conversation? Should we only accept men with spotless records as allies? Can we trust heterosexual men to speak honestly, and not just use the movement as cover? Do we, ultimately, believe it's possible for them to change?"

These are pressing questions for men who have inherited the privileges of structural injustice while claiming the "spotless record." My instinctive response, in the face of white-hot female rage, is silence and submission. If my time's up, the floor is yours. I am quick to shut up. If I am irredeemably implicated by my advantages, and the willingness to change is not the same as the capacity to change, then I am the first to get out of the way.

Yet if Hill and others believed an effective way forward is for all men to move aside and STFU, then she would have said so. Instead, she promotes the idea that for change to be ongoing, coalitions must be built and maintained.

Many years ago, I met Nina Funnell when she was in the early days of her work to expose and end sexual abuse on university campuses. I offered help. If I have dedicated my writing career to the defeat of a single adversary (never underestimate the importance of revenge in a writer's motivations), my nemesis can be portrayed succinctly – and Jess Hill does so at the heart of her essay – as my personal Christian Porter. Through satire, extended analysis in fiction and nonfiction, every means possible. I have given a life to exposing such men, in the somewhat optimistic hope of bringing about some kind of self-recognition and reflection. If you like, Funnell and I had the same target in our sights.

Of course, she didn't need my help. She had the testimony of thousands of women who had their own young Christian Porters. And while I was, I hoped, holding such men to account for their subtler abuses and their blind habitation of their glittering burrows, Funnell was potentially uncovering actual crimes. As a male observing toxic masculinity, as someone whose sufferings were relatively minor, I could only go so far.

So should the male voice, with his privileges and impending decrepitude, simply box up his good intentions and vanish? In many ways, it would be a relief. It has never been as easy as it is now to be misunderstood, and when you are misread and anathematised by your friends and allies, the overwhelming temptation is to curl up in a ball and be silent.

Yet shutting up and submitting, being too humble, not challenging forceful personalities, yielding the floor – this was what my kind did in the first place. It was our part in letting our Christian Porters do what they did. Fear of confrontation, fear of power and fear of ridicule lay behind our complicity in their acts. Silence and withdrawal by the many is what enables crimes by the few. Male passivity doesn't get as much coverage as active violence, but is one of the (in)actions that got us here.

Hill co-wrote her final chapter with her husband, David Hollier. She accepts Josh Bornstein's first-person plural pronoun when he asks, "Are we winning?" This ought to clarify the message for men who consider themselves innocent and yet still guilty, who wonder if the best thing they can do is to be silent. The "unceasing" battle that Hill describes in her conclusion can be fought in many ways, but she suggests that it can only be won by working together.

Malcolm Knox

Janet Albrechtsen

The Reckoning is, on many levels, a terrific analysis of the #MeToo movement in this country and elsewhere. Jess Hill lays down an excellent timeline of how #MeToo started with waves of rage and retribution in October 2017, radiating from a hashtag to where it landed in Australia at the clumsy feet of Scott Morrison by the end of 2021. In between, Hill covers the disaster of the early days of #MeToo in Australia when Tracey Spicer made "impossible promises" of a "triage service" to help women. Hill also offers sensible analysis of the need to focus on the long game of embedding cultural change to protect all women from abuse, rather than just the Whack-a-Mole wins against high-profile men.

What's missing from Hill's essay is a greater understanding of why many have been frustrated by and disappointed with the exploitation of the #MeToo movement. For example, Hill regards the sceptical reaction of Germaine Greer and other older feminists to #MeToo as a "surprising twist."

Why surprising? Not every claim under the #MeToo banner deserved, or deserves, to be taken seriously. Not all women are powerless patsies in the workplace.

Hill's essay would have been more compelling if the messy, wondrous complexities of men and women and their sexual relationships got a run. Instead, it repeats the #MeToo pattern of treating us as simpletons, unable to agree to cultural change unless women are seen as powerless victims and masculinity as inherently bad, a road that takes our boys to confusion, misogyny and abuse.

Many women hold power in the workplace. Some abuse it. Women can manipulate men sexually and emotionally. Women can choose to have sexual relationships with powerful bosses without a scintilla of regret. Some will do it deliberately to climb the career ladder. In some cases, it's the thundering power of love between two people who happen to work in the same place. Sometimes the love is uneven, and when there is no marriage proposal, all hell breaks loose into claims of abuse. Who holds the power in that scenario?

Hill's Quarterly Essay would have benefited from more curiosity, perhaps even bravery, to explore how the #MeToo movement has ensnared – and been co-opted by – many people for purposes beyond abuse and male power.

Take the front-page headline in London's *Daily Mail* about Meghan Markle on 7 January 2022: "'Bullying' is word used to harm career women, says Meghan's lawyer." Maybe sometimes. The word does get thrown around a lot when women fall out with colleagues. But not always. Women can be terrible bullies, as data from the latest report into the federal parliament's culture shows.

If we are serious about cultural change, honesty is the best policy. That means recognising the good, the bad and the ugly in men and women.

Janet Albrechtsen

This response was first published in *The Australian* on 7 January 2022.

Kieran Pender

The Reckoning is contemporary history – the first account of seismic developments that will continue to be dissected for decades to come. The essay does an excellent job of explaining and assessing. But understandably, it only begins the task of answering the critical question: what do we do about it? It is this question I want to consider. It is an urgent one, because, as Hill acknowledges, "consciousness-raising movements have for fifty years revealed the ubiquity of sexual harassment." We should not be so naive as to think that change is inevitable, or that we will inevitably succeed where our predecessors failed. If we want a society in which sexual harassment is vanishingly rare, not drearily commonplace, in which women feel safe and respected, not coerced, abused and harassed, we must address Australia's harassment epidemic.

The first, trite thing to say is that there is no panacea. Sexual harassment in the workplace, in education and in social life generally is a complex phenomenon, as is its twin, domestic and family abuse. It is no wonder that the *Respect@Work* report is 932 pages long and contains fifty-five recommendations. Preventing and addressing sexual harassment in all spheres of life will take a blend of education, law reform, funding and initiatives ranging from innovative to mundane, from governments and non-government stakeholders alike.

It has been heartening to see increasingly sophisticated public discourse around these issues, and Labor's promise to implement the outstanding *Respect@Work* recommendations if elected. However, much media attention has focused on particular recommendations, such as the proposed positive duty on employers to take reasonable and proportionate measures to prevent workplace sexual harassment. We should be wary of fixating on single solutions. I share the optimism of both Hill and Josh Bornstein, who variously describe the proposal – championed by Sex Discrimination Commissioner Kate Jenkins – as "revolutionary" and "potentially game-changing." But a new legislative provision alone will not cause cultural change.

Focusing on particular interventions is tempting but undesirable because cultural change is messy. We progress and we regress; it is not always possible to identify what causes change and what contributes to resistance. We cannot A/B test efforts to address deep-seated social problems. Placing a positive duty on employers and adopting Jenkins' other suggestions for funding and reform are necessary, but not sufficient, components of change. They are the start, not the end, of the journey.

Perhaps the most difficult piece in this jigsaw puzzle is the role of men. As Hill rightly observes, these are issues not of women's safety, but of men's violence. To effectively address the prevalence and impact of sexual harassment in Australian life, we have to fix men. This point has a few dimensions.

It is a necessary corollary that if sexual harassment is rife in Australian society, then so too are sexual harassers. My 2019 research for the International Bar Association, the peak global body for the legal profession, found that one in three female lawyers had been sexually harassed at work (the number in Australia was even higher). As we know from the Australian Human Rights Commission, cited by Hill, a similar proportion of Australians has been sexually harassed across all workplaces within the past five years.

Most interested observers will be aware of these or similar figures. But what we have not fully confronted is the consequence: that a similar percentage of male lawyers, and Australian men, have committed sexual harassment at work. I say "similar," not "the same," because there are no doubt serial perpetrators who harass many times. Even so, hundreds of thousands of Australian men have committed sexual harassment. That is not a wild aspersion, but a clear statistical inference. There are over 13 million Australians in the workforce, and, according to the AHRC, over four million of those have been sexually harassed in the past five years. Consider, as a rough estimate, that the average perpetrator harassed four people in that time: this would mean one million Australians have perpetrated sexual harassment in recent years. One million sexual harassers. Almost all are men.

The second point is that many, probably most, of those one million harassers are not the archetypal perpetrator. They are not Harvey Weinstein or Dyson Heydon – unrepentant wrongdoers who deserve opprobrium, but who are also easy fallguys for wider social sins. Instead, they are all around us: our fathers, brothers, friends.

Most sexual harassment is not of the kind committed by Weinstein and Heydon. The AHRC's most recent national prevalence survey found that sexually suggestive comments or jokes, intrusive questions about a person's private life and inappropriate staring were the most common forms of workplace sexual harassment. Inappropriate physical conduct was less frequent (experienced by 9 per cent of survey respondents), while just 1 per cent had experienced sexual assault.

I say this not to minimise those other forms of conduct, which can have an equally significant negative impact on the target of the harassment – whether as an individual incident or pattern of behaviour. All sexual harassment is wrong and unlawful; some is also criminal. But by focusing on the high-profile cases – at the more severe end of the spectrum of conduct – we risk obscuring the pervasive, everyday and, dare I say, "ordinary" sexual harassment. We make it too easy for the million-odd perpetrators to think: "I'm not Harvey Weinstein, I'm not the problem." The typical perpetrator is not a bogeyman. It is you, or me.

If the #MeToo movement is to succeed, in Australia and elsewhere, it must address these everyday experiences of sexual harassment. This is no easy task. In individual workplaces, and in civil and criminal law, clear accountability mechanisms exist for serious forms of sexual harassment (even if too many workplaces still wish to conceal rather than address incidents). But what of the grey areas – the sexual joke in the elevator, the possibly suggestive text from a boss to their staff member, the colleague leaning in for an unreciprocated kiss at after-work drinks? In these contexts, right and wrong are not always as clearly distinguished – subtle cues, power dynamics and subjective interpretation can be everything.

It is in these contexts that the million Australian perpetrators can mainly be found – not committing Weinstein-esque behaviour, but making inappropriate comments, or being "too friendly". It is still sexual harassment, but it is not the type that will be addressed by blunt legislative instruments. We can improve sexual harassment laws, fund more and better support, and require employers to take preventative and responsive action. But addressing such "ordinary," everyday harassment requires cultural change: it requires us to fix men.

How? I don't claim to have all the answers. Education – starting in kindergarten or earlier – has a big role to play. Above all, cultural change requires pragmatism. It necessitates constructive engagement with half of the population. Some men – the Weinsteins – might never change. For them, we need accountability. But for the rest, we need engagement, conversations, patience and space.

I appreciate that it is easy for a man to say this. I have never been sexually harassed. I understand the righteous anger. It should not be up to women to fix men. While anger is helpful in driving accountability, we need more than anger to ensure enduring change. I thought Hill's passage about Richie Hardcore, a New

Zealand martial arts champion engaging with men to address misogyny, was instructive: "What use is being 'right' if we end up alienating the very men we want to listen to us, and change?"

This is the paradox of #MeToo. The movement represented a seismic opportunity for women to break decades of silence; to finally speak their truth and be heard. But we need to engage men in the conversation if we are to move from consciousness-raising to cultural change. Engaging men does not mean taking power away from women. It does not mean handing over the microphone. But it does mean speaking, and listening, in safe spaces, accepting that people come with different perspectives and different language, and might be at different places on the learning curve.

That might sound unpalatable: it should be enough that men listen and then change their ways. Yet it is not. It is therefore unpalatable, but necessary, for both women and men to engage men on these issues. Men have a special responsibility – to call out poor behaviour, to educate one another, to be good allies. But, however frustrating, we cannot rely on men alone to fix men. It may be tempting, not unreasonably so in the face of millennia of patriarchal oppression, to be righteous. We will achieve change by being pragmatic.

The final page of *The Reckoning* makes for sobering reading. Hill quotes Faludi: "Declaring war is thrilling. Nation-building isn't." Hill then adds: "But the job will never be done ... There is no utopia waiting for us. We make the gains while we can, we celebrate the advances, and then we get back to work." This is a sentiment I have tried to impart many times during my work campaigning to address harassment in the legal profession. This is a campaign like no other, because there is no finish line. We will never get to harassment zero. But that does not mean we should not try.

Everyone has a right to feel safe, supported and respected, at all times and in all spaces. To go some way towards achieving that, we must get back to work. This is a task in which every single Australian has a role to play, men especially.

Kieran Pender

Sara Dowse

Two pages into the introduction of Jess Hill's Quarterly Essay is a sentence that jumped off the page at me: "But then things get dark." She was referring to what happened after Prime Minister Scott Morrison revealed in a highly emotional statement to the press gallery that, despite his dissembling and shelving of the issue for weeks, he had come to learn what it's been like for women, throughout Australia and in the very building where he was standing.

First, a few remarks about Morrison's statement. It came after months of mounting anger as the #MeToo wave had crashed with full force into Parliament House – the centre, as is often said, of Australian democracy. On the Ides of March, women all over the country had spilled into the streets in a March 4 Justice and in Canberra they rallied on the Parliament House lawn. Putting it mildly, parliamentary workplace behaviour had been found wanting. A woman had been allegedly raped in the defence minister's office, only a few feet from Morrison's own. A male staffer had been photographed by his mates while jerking off onto a female MP's desk. The attorney-general had outed himself as the accused in a historical case of alleged rape. Morrison seemed to have finally grasped that a deep-seated misogyny runs through our nation, finding its most horrific expression in what can only be called a scourge of sexual violence.

#MeToo has reminded us that misogyny – or sexism, as we termed it in the 1970s – operates systemically. At the milder end of the spectrum are the put-downs, the mansplaining, the crude remarks. Then come the unwanted sexual advances that can morph into outright harassment. *But then things get dark* – the endgame being sexual assault and all too often murder.

In the corporate world at least, strides have been made to lessen the incidence of sexual harassment in the workplace, which is illegal under the 1984 *Sex Discrimination Act*. In this respect, as Hill proceeds to skilfully outline, parliament is an egregious outlier, a world unto its own. For all Morrison's histrionics at the press conference – about how the women in his life constitute its centre, and that because of them he was going to *do* something – the prime minister reverted to form. To the suggestion from a News Corp reporter that he might have lost control of his staff, the PM lashed back with an insinuation about an incident alleged to have occurred in a Sky News toilet. As Hill explains, there was no such incident. It is this "mask-dropping", coded retort that Hill alludes to with her *But then things get dark*.

I'm not here to repeat what Hill explains about this gaffe and what it reveals about Morrison. For me, her simple five-word sentence has far greater resonance. It encapsulates the dismayingly cyclical nature of what one prescient writer in the '70s called "the longest revolution." Feminism's progress – and it *is* progress – has been glacially slow. Now and then it gathers swift momentum, until it lands like a meteorite on the body politic. Such was the force of the suffragist movement. Then it was left to simmer, buried under the post-war patriarchal resurgence of the 1950s, until it burst out again. And each time it bursts out, as it did again in the 1970s, the women caught up in it experience a thrillingly cathartic exhilaration, as the justice of the cause becomes so bleedingly obvious.

And then things get dark.

I'm talking about backlash. It's not surprising that Hill ends her magnificent essay by confronting it. "A century from now, women will be holding signs," she affirms, "just as they did at the March 4 Justice – that say 'I can't believe we're still protesting this shit.'" She even suggests that, as successful as it has been in effecting cultural change through exposing and rooting out misogyny in the entertainment and legal worlds, #MeToo appears to have triggered its own backlash. Writing this on the brink of a federal election, after all that's been shown to be morally threadbare in Morrison's idea of governance, I find this cause for concern. From what we know about him now, he will not be pitching for votes from feminists or our supporters, but from those in whom our own special brand of Australian misogyny has been left to fester and ominously sprout.

Yet there's another way of looking at it. In the 1970s, when feminism's second wave reached us here in Australia, we women found enough homegrown grievances to make the movement our own. Where to begin? Jobs advertised along gender lines. "Public" bars closed to women. Unequal pay inscribed in industry awards and cemented in a basic minimum wage. Childcare was scarce and substandard. There was a luxury tax on contraceptives; abortion was illegal and highly dangerous. There were no women bus drivers, let alone pilots. We scarcely made an appearance in the law faculties, not to mention the High Court. Not a single woman occupied a seat in the House of Representatives. You never heard or saw a woman reading the news or providing commentary. With staggeringly few exceptions, all positions of authority were reserved for males, for underpinning it all was the pervasive, peculiarly Australian patriarchal culture that effectively consigned half the adult population to second-class citizenship. It's hard even for women (like me) who were alive back then to grasp how we were treated, and unimaginable to my daughters and granddaughters. But for all that, it could be said we were lucky, because feminism's resurgence coincided with the 1972 election of a federal government prepared to put energy and resources into improving the situation. And it was a shift in the hitherto conservative women's vote that put them there.

In the three tumultuous years that Whitlam was allowed to govern, the changes to Australian society were both remarkable and long-lasting. That doesn't mean that no one resisted them or that reform came easily. But if the momentum slowed after the 1975 Dismissal, it picked up again after 1983, when Labor was returned. It was only with the Coalition's election under Howard in 1996 that women took a slide, and things became steadily darker. Women in politics were more visible than they had been, a female MP was no longer an oddity, there were women in the ministry, a few made it into cabinet. But Howard's brand of conservatism was marked by a nostalgic yearning for the 1950s, and key measures of his government, such as the family tax benefit part B and Costello's baby bonus, were imbued with it. This was the "post-feminist" era. Women were induced to become "homemakers" again, and what feminism remained was narrowly interpreted as "leaning in," or middle-class career advancement, or abstruse academic theory. The cost of childcare rocketed; the effective marginal tax rate on married women lowered the female participation rate, leaving many older women today with insufficient superannuation to fund their retirements. Correspondingly, cuts to women's refuges and associated services left women unacceptably vulnerable.

Yet throughout this, the "post-feminist" claptrap and Howard's social conservatism, one crucial change from those earlier, heady reformist years survived. Enough of what we second-wave feminists had achieved had rubbed off on younger women – even those who shunned the designation. Greater education opportunity had a part in it. For all Howard's efforts, women had wider aspirations for themselves and were bound to be enraged when thwarted, meeting up with glass ceilings, sexual harassment and violence. Here was a classic case of approach-suppression – the kind that makes for revolutions.

It's possible that, after the decades of backlash, the hideous treatment dished out to our one female prime minister and worse to countless other women, and the whittling away of essential government services, women will prove crucial in voting out a government that has shown itself particularly impervious to our concerns. Could it be time – once again?

Maybe it should come as no surprise that at the time of writing eight out of the eleven independents seeking to win previously safe Coalition seats in the coming election happen to be women. I live in Warringah, where we are bracing ourselves for what the Liberals will unleash in attempting to wrest the seat back. They were as dirty as hell in 2019 trying to stop Zali Steggall from getting elected. We're not complacent, we know the tricks the Liberals are capable of. But the signs are that Steggall will be re-elected. She's proved an intelligent, hardworking and responsive member, and the issues she's fought for, in the 2019 campaign and subsequently in parliament, are of increasing urgency in the electorate. Climate change is one, integrity another. Feminism is another. At one event I attended back in 2019, the moderator, Layne Beachley, asked what had prompted Steggall to run. Steggall didn't hesitate with an answer. It was seeing how the Liberals treated Julie Bishop in the spill that elected Morrison, she said, dropping Bishop off early in the ballot in favour of a man – any man. And needless to say, Steggall is no fan of Morrison.

The election this year is expected to be the most important in a generation – on the order of 1972's – though even if history does repeat itself, the script is never quite the same. The overriding issue in the 1970s was our involvement in Vietnam, and Labor had promised to withdraw our troops. (Imagine how it would be wedged on something comparable today.) For women, the "mandate" included opening the case for equal pay and funding for preschools (though not for childcare). The Women's Electoral Lobby's questionnaire was significant in raising awareness of what were called "women's issues" and exposing how ignorant of them some of the candidates were, most notably the sitting prime minister, Billy McMahon.

We've yet to see if the #MeToo groundswell will translate into enough votes for the female independents to gain the balance of power in the forty-seventh parliament, or if the women's vote per se will be the deciding factor in a Labor victory, as it was in 1972. Certainly the incompetence, "soft" corruption and generally vacuous management of Morrison and his ministers provide reason enough for their losing women's votes.

Hill rightly ends her essay on a note of cautious optimism. "We are winning the war," she writes. Yet she also warns that the success of #MeToo, this latest iteration in feminism's "longest revolution," has set off its own backlash, one resulting in a deepening electoral gender divide, at the centre of which could be climate change – already deemed by some to be a "feminine" issue. And if Omicron peters out by election day, Morrison's infuriating stunts playing to his toxic male "base" could just possibly save him. That said, I wouldn't put my money on it. Things have got far too dark.

Sara Dowse

Nareen Young

Jess Hill's essay is a necessary, if at times exhausting, retelling and analysis of the recent post-#MeToo years. I agree with her conclusion that while some battles are being lost, the war is being won. I see this as a long-term project – there is so much more to be done.

As a feminist of both Aboriginal and culturally diverse descent, I agree with Tracy Westerman's succinct tweet of 27 January 2022: "I want to see #MeToo champion Aboriginal victims, particularly given its black origins & the invisibility of Aboriginal victims." My characterisation of the Australian version of #MeToo as an individualist, white, corporate feminist–centred problem lacking focus on structural reform is well known, as Hill recounts, but that's not to say that I think we should cease our efforts to create much-needed change.

Having been a workplace legal practitioner for many years, I feel the next big battle is placing a positive duty on employers to prevent sexual harassment. This is "unfinished business." This critical recommendation from Kate Jenkins' work cannot be lost if we are to make real progress in the workplace.

The statistics on harassment in the workplace are both shocking and unsurprising, given the lived experience of so many women. As a former director of the NSW Working Women's Centre, I am intimately familiar with this lived experience. Finishing off the "unfinished business" should involve the proper funding of referral pathways, especially the Working Women's Centres (also a recommendation of the Jenkins review).

Nearly five years on from #MeToo going viral, it is a sad reflection of the very slow pace of progress that we are only now getting such basic change and support for victims. The Morrison government has just announced that sexual harassment will be added to 1800Respect's remit, but it is still unclear if the Working Women's Centres will be properly resourced to deal with the influx. We know growing awareness of different forms of gendered violence always leads to more "help seeking," and it would be a scandal of a different order if the Morrison government raised victims' hopes that help is there, only to disappoint them.

All this is to illustrate that there are so many issues and changes we need to track and continue to fight for collectively. And that's long after the mainstream media band moves on, or white corporate feminists who claim "the movement" as their own, then gate-keep and co-opt it for their own ends (activism is collective, not part of anyone's "brand"), lose interest.

Anyone who thinks changing a few HR policies will bring true change is kidding themselves. I'm sorry to say that in so many cases, I have observed HR to be the friend of the company, not of the victim of harassment. It is too often the case that making a complaint actually makes the situation worse. A positive duty to prevent harassment would be a legal obligation producing more immediate and effective change than a thousand HR policies.

Whatever the outcome of the next election, the next government needs to be held to account to ensure full implementation of Kate Jenkins' recommendations.

Nareen Young

Jess Hill

Before I respond to the correspondence, I'd like to apologise to ABC journalist Louise Milligan for an error I made in the essay. Milligan did not, as I wrote, contact the late Kate Thornton's lawyer, Michael Bradley, after being tipped off by Kate's friend Nick Ryan. She was given that information by another (confidential) source. Nick Ryan had nothing to do with Milligan discovering that Christian Porter was the subject of these allegations.

The mood at the National Press Club on 9 February was tense and electric and anxious and generous. Journalist, advocates, politicians and – at every table – women who had survived sexual violence. Reckless hugging. Old comrades reunited.

We were gathered and waiting for an address from two young women, Brittany Higgins and Grace Tame, who had fixed the nation's attention on sexual violence, and the government's failure to respond to it. Battle-hardened feminists were nervous for the two women in the green room upstairs giving their speeches one last read. Would Australia – a country run mostly by mates and blokes – really let these two young women define this cultural moment? Or would their words end up being twisted and misrepresented? Would this be the moment two victim-survivors set the agenda for this election year – and the years ahead – or would it set in train a silencing backlash?

Since I finished writing Quarterly Essay 84, something has shifted again. After a year of public reckoning over sexual violence – which the Morrison government presumed to be a temporary flashpoint best handled with spin and patience – the heat has not abated. In fact, the cultural power of victim-survivors has only grown. In January, when Tame had the audacity to show the prime minister how she felt about him – stony-faced and side-eyed at the Lodge, fulfilling her last duties as Australian of the Year – hers was the face that launched a thousand columns. It wasn't "civil," it wasn't "nice," she was doing what women had been warned against for millennia, she was a feminist hero – within hours, she went from a public figure to an icon, photoshopped onto five-dollar notes as Australia's larrikin queen.

This is a new kind of power – and an unprecedented change, I believe, in the way Western societies have traditionally regarded victim-survivors of sexual violence. If I was to get carried away (if I had a column to write, let's say), I might look at this cultural transformation and see in it a historic paradigmatic shift – one that is seeing some victim-survivors imbued for the first time with power, wisdom and expertise. I can't name a time in the history of Western civilisation in which this has been the case; for millennia, victim-survivors have been pitied (at best), blamed, shamed, pathologised and ostracised. Even in Greek mythology, rape survivors are expected to accept their lot. It's in Indigenous stories that we find historical examples of this "new" paradigm: "The Tale of the Raped Maiden," for example, in which a twenty-year-old Ojibwe woman is, in the wake of being abducted and raped by a warring tribe, welcomed back by her own people as a wise and powerful woman who becomes both a medicine woman and a warrior.

There's nothing wrong with trying to take a bird's-eye view of this cultural moment, to place it in a historical context and assess what it may portend. But it's easy to get carried away and disconnect our analysis from the real lives of the people we're writing about. The more important point to make – and perhaps what is central to her appeal – is that Tame herself is not the property of a single movement, she is not angling to be an icon and she is not ideological. As she tweeted in response to the Australian of the Year furore, "What I did wasn't an act of martyrdom in the gender culture war. It's true that many women are sick of being told to smile, often by men, for the benefit of men. But it's not just women who are conditioned to smile and conform to the visibly rotting status quo. It's all of us."

When Tame stood behind the lectern at the National Press Club in February, she said a lot, and with such presence and conviction that it was almost impossible to look away. What I jotted down, while I still had the presence of mind to take notes, were not the lines that ended up dominating headlines later that day. They were lines in her speech that spoke directly to a marginalised cohort of people watching at home; lines that may offer us a chance to find common ground, and to stop sexual violence being described reductively as a "women's issue." She was standing there not as a victim of sexual assault, "which is a distinctly gendered issue," but as a target of child sexual abuse.

"I am not just an advocate for women," she said. "I am an advocate for all survivors of child sexual abuse, many of whom are male." The need to preserve the distinction between sexual assault (which predominantly affects women) and child sexual abuse (which disproportionately affects girls, but also affects a significant percentage of boys) was crucial, she continued. "We cannot forget our boys, and we cannot forget our men, not only as welcome, equal participants in this ongoing conversation, and without ignoring many negative patriarchal customs, we cannot forget our boys and men who are fellow survivors of abuse."

Tame was throwing down the gauntlet to the women's movement: Can we broaden this conversation to include the boys and men who have been subjected to sexual violence and abuse? Domestic abuse, sexual violence and child sexual abuse differ in important ways, but, as Tame said, they are all about abuse of power. "Men are not the enemy," she said. "Abuse of power is the enemy." Men make up the overwhelming majority of perpetrators, especially of sexual violence, but this resistance to advocating for survivor boys and men must be overcome. The target of the feminist movement made more precise: abusers of power, upholders of patriarchy.

Since Rosie Batty was made Australian of the Year in 2015, we've spent years as a nation interrogating the nature of abuse and violence, and have dramatically recalibrated our attitudes to, and beliefs about, victim-survivors. In this conversation, however – still – the perpetrators are largely invisible, and often misunderstood. This issue remains, as Kieran Pender writes in his correspondence, "perhaps the most difficult piece in this jigsaw puzzle [of solutions]." What do we do with the hundreds of thousands – if not millions – of men who harass, abuse, coerce and control? When will people truly internalise the reality that the men who do the most damage aren't just those who commit the obvious dastardly acts – the Harvey Weinsteins and Dyson Heydons – but "our fathers, brothers, friends ... The typical perpetrator is not a bogeyman. It is you, or me." That is a paradigm shift which is yet to take root in this country. That's understandable: the idea that the men we love and treasure could be behaving in ways we find repugnant is deeply unsettling. But if we don't grapple with this – while taking care not to demonise men in general – we will continue to misdiagnose both the problem and the solutions.

In his thought-provoking response, Pender also highlights the need to reconceive what constitutes the greater harm when it comes to sexual harassment. We are, as a society, preoccupied with blockbuster incidents, and find it much harder to comprehend the extreme harm done through objectification and degradation. "What of the grey areas – the sexual joke in the elevator, the possibly suggestive text from a boss to their staff member, the colleague leaning in for an unreciprocated kiss at after-work drinks? In these contexts, right and wrong are not always so clearly distinguished – subtle cues, power dynamics and subjective interpretation can be everything ... If the #MeToo movement is to succeed, in Australia and elsewhere, it must address these everyday experiences of sexual harassment." My own experience of sexual harassment, which I detailed in the essay, was not a headline-making incident – it was a blunt kind of sexual objectification. And yet, more than fifteen years later, writing about it brought back such powerful feelings of worthlessness that I was left sobbing at my desk.

I won't speak for women of previous generations, but I can say that I believe my response was heavily influenced by the fact that I didn't grow up with any sense that my gender would affect – let alone define – the way I would be treated in the workplace. In fact, although I was disturbed as a teenager by the way women were talked down to in fashion magazines, it took me another decade to realise that this was symptomatic of the broader system of gender inequality. So when, in my early twenties, I was sexually objectified by my boss (several decades my senior), it shattered the innate sense I had of being entitled to equal treatment. It initiated me into a world I had no idea existed.

Since *The Reckoning* was published, three young former associates sexually harassed by former High Court judge Dyson Heydon finally received their settlement, reported to be a six-figure sum, from the Morrison government. Asked by Laura Tingle on 7.30 if she had anything she'd like to tell Heydon, one of those associates, Alex Eggerking, summed up with cold fury and precision the life-altering harm of being coerced and sexually objectified by one of the country's most senior judges. "Dyson, you ruined my career. You destroyed my love for the law … You made me feel viscerally unsafe on my third day of working for you. You made me feel worthless. You treated me like I was an object that you could use when you wanted to with impunity." She went on: "What I also want to say is that you didn't get away with it. Strong, courageous, vulnerable, bloody determined women stood up and said, 'That's enough. This is what happened to me and you won't get away with it.'" The fury and indignation of women like Eggerking (and so many others whose names we have learnt since 2017), who were raised to expect equality, is the lifeblood of #MeToo and this powerful era of modern feminism.

Apparently, however, Janet Albrechtsen doesn't share their indignation. Having said that, it's unclear whether Albrechtsen read the whole essay. She is a culture warrior, first and foremost, which tends to preclude close engagement on issues within the battlelines. When she says "not all women are powerless patsies in the workplace," it's unclear to whom she is referring. Are the women who were involuntarily conscripted into #MeToo in Australia, simply through making a complaint, "powerless patsies"? Are women who *don't* complain, by extension, powerful and independent? Should women just cop it and not make a fuss? Does Albrechtsen consider sexual harassment an unavoidable (albeit unfortunate) feature of working life for women? The mind boggles.

For this essay, I wrote 40,000 words in seven weeks (with the invaluable assistance of David Hollier and Kristine Ziwica), and I readily concede that I could not do justice to every aspect of the #MeToo movement. But nowhere on my list of subjects to include did I have the "messy, wondrous complexities of men and women and their sexual relationships." My subject was #MeToo, which is concerned with sexual violence. I took it as given that readers know the difference between complex relationships and patterns of sexual harassment, coercion, assault and rape. Of course, the lines are not always precise, but my essay is concerned with behaviour that falls well outside the spectrum of "wondrous" and crosses over into "traumatising" and "illegal." If Albrechtsen is suggesting that more analysis is needed of the grey areas regarding consent, I would direct her to chapter two, in which the Aziz Ansari case illustrates just that. In fact, clarifying these boundaries makes "wondrous" relationships more likely, not less.

Albrechtsen also suggests that the essay "would have benefited from more curiosity, perhaps even bravery, to explore how the #MeToo movement has ensnared – and been co-opted by – many people for purposes beyond abuse and male power." I'm curious: which cases would exemplify this? Who has co-opted the movement? Albrechtsen is not explicit – or should I say, she does not appear curious enough herself here to give examples. In my work on gendered violence, I err towards challenging the status quo – for example, the accepted wisdom that gender inequality is at the root of domestic abuse (and is therefore an effective way to address it). I have never shied away from tipping a sacred cow on its head and examining its parts. But aside from analysing this as a hypothetical, I genuinely do not know what Albrechtsen would have me analyse – what credible example of #MeToo being co-opted or abused I would single out as a reflection of a broader dynamic. I don't see how, on the evidence, #MeToo has led to a pattern of men being ensnared by false allegations.

It would be nice if Albrechtsen at some point acknowledged Australia's endemic and, by international standards, very high rates of serious abuse of power in the forms of sexual harassment, assault and rape in workplaces and elsewhere. In fact, in Australia's legal profession – to which Albrechtsen claims membership – harassment and abuse are so common they have long been accepted as part of the culture, a rite of passage for many. I wonder if Albrechtsen considers sexual harassment an inevitable, even normal, part of career advancement for women.

I am grateful for the cool-headed analysis of my journalistic peers, particularly Gina Rushton, Hannah Ryan and Amber Schultz. Rushton and Ryan are right to carve up my optimistic conclusion into quantifiable chunks: Exactly how can we tell if we are winning this war? Can we see actual change in how allegations are received? Whether sexual harassment has diminished? Aside from relaying anecdotal evidence, it's impossible to answer these questions with any confidence. Journalist and survivor advocate Nina Funnell has cautioned against overblown optimism, particularly that which centred on the Women's March in 2021. Momentum that is not bedded down in real reform can easily be lost, and to paraphrase the great Harvard psychiatrist Judith Herman, "trauma wants to be forgotten." Perhaps rather than try to assess change through the shorter lens of the immediate past, it's more helpful to zoom out, to see how similarly powerful movements have brought about historic change – the kind of change we now take for granted. Here, I defer to the correspondence of feminist and author Sara Dowse, who has had a front-row seat to many of the changes that preceded #MeToo, to give us a sense of what is possible.

Yet, of all the seismic changes we have seen since Dowse was a young woman, what we have not seen elevated in this movement is the equal inclusion of Indigenous women and women of colour. This was made painfully clear in the wake of the government's hastily organised apology to those who had experienced sexual harassment, assault or bullying while working in federal parliament – an occasion to which the government did not deem it necessary to invite any of the women it was apologising to. Instead, a small number of survivors and advocates was hastily invited at the last minute, thanks to the intervention of independent MP Zali Steggall. There were several there, such as Chanel Contos, who had not worked in the parliament, and yet still, however, nobody thought to invite women of colour such as Dhanya Mani, a former NSW Liberal political staffer who went public with her allegations of sexual assault by a colleague, or Tessa Sullivan, who was the first political staffer to have their allegations made public after #MeToo, as readers of the essay will recall. Mani's objections to this ongoing erasure were read out in parliament by Queensland Greens MP Larissa Waters:

"Even now in 2022, after the lessons of #MeToo, politicians and the mainstream media almost solely centre the stories of cisgender, able-bodied and conventionally attractive white women at the expense of all other voices. But this cultural moment of reckoning in Australian politics and feminism is built on the sacrifice, advocacy and unpaid labour of women of colour like me. Like Tessa. We came first."

Nareen Young highlights this inexcusable disparity in her correspondence, citing a comment that speaks to the necessity of this change: "As a feminist of both Aboriginal and culturally diverse descent, I agree with Tracy Westerman's succinct tweet of 27 January 2022 that 'I want to see #MeToo champion Aboriginal victims, particularly given its Black origins & the invisibility of Aboriginal victims.'"

We need to shift the dial on this, and quickly, lest we embed just another archetype of the "ideal victim."

We are living through one of those peak times, when, as Dowse writes, the "justice of the cause" has become "so bleedingly obvious" – but perhaps for the first time not just to women, but also to a growing number of men. There is something quite astonishing about the appeal of Brittany Higgins and Grace Tame to a growing number of men who are impressed by their chutzpah and do not feel excluded by their rhetoric. It is clear who attracts their ire: those who abuse power. As Higgins made so devastatingly clear in her address to the National Press Club: "I did not want his sympathy as a father; I wanted him to use his power as prime minister." These are appeals not to empathy and compassion, but to a clarity of ethics and leadership. This is a message that is resonating with a growing cohort of men, who can see a shared vision in their words. So how can supportive men become part of the change they want to see in the world?

This is addressed somewhat in Malcolm Knox's genuine and heartfelt response. I hand the mic over here to my partner, psychotherapist David Hollier, who co-wrote the essay's chapter on men:

"Malcom Knox's response plumbs the exact position of this essay on men's response to the demands of #MeToo: listen, understand, stay engaged, work together. As a psychotherapist, I have worked with many men grappling with problems rooted in their experiences of being male; I can attest that Knox is not alone in feeling that 'silence and submission' is the smartest response to #MeToo. Faced with social media that so readily distort and weaponise even well-intentioned, considered contributions, too many men fall into the passivity that Knox rightly identifies as collusion. Every man must ask himself how it is that women need a movement to demand, to plead with us not to harass, assault and rape them. Start by facing the absurd notion that this is, still, apparently, an unrealistic request.

"As one of three men who along with sixty-odd women participated in UNSW's inaugural gender studies class in 1995, I've long since thought feminism has as much, and in the long run more, to offer men than women; but for men to shed the skin of patriarchal, power-over masculinity requires a far more threatening metamorphosis, one that requires trust, the courage to let one's guard down long enough to connect on terms of shared power. I have found that simply discussing this with men draws a threat response from many, a reaction that is more deeply embedded, more primal, more rapidly aroused, than anything in our cognition – men's mistrust of men. Most feel a loss of control and fear before they can reach the relief of discovering they can let their guard down and still be okay. Just writing these words, I brace for the onslaught of reactive defensiveness, the excuses that invariably follow the offer of connection. Here is where men must encourage and support each other, shed the defences.

"As a therapist, I challenge men in the safety of a confidential closed room, men who have chosen to ask questions about their masculinity and the damaging effects it has on their lives – their families and friends. From this private space, I thank Knox and the many other men who have risked men's – and some women's – opprobrium when they have dared to publicly challenge the old-world masculinity and privilege so stubbornly abiding in Australia. May such voices proliferate."

Finally, although the apology – snuck in the day before the address by Tame and Higgins to the National Press Club – was another impeccably designed PR disaster, I'm interested in what it says about the loose ends Morrison perceives as a threat to his re-election – it's not enough just to play the buffoon to the blokes and the patient women who love them. The "issues" that women have with men's violence may not decide the election, but they are clearly enough of a worry to see the government now give priority to the response – both to the internal Jenkins report and, theatrically, with the apology. Being faced with a slew of mostly female independents in marginal seats must also have sharpened the Coalition's attention. It seems women may be sufficiently disgusted by this government to change their vote. How many women? We'll have the answer by the time the next Quarterly Essay is published.

Jess Hill

Janet Albrechtsen is an opinion columnist with *The Australian*. She has worked as a solicitor in commercial law and holds a doctorate of juridical studies from the University of Sydney.

Sara Dowse led the Office of Women's Affairs under Gough Whitlam and Malcolm Fraser, developing policy for federal funding of women's services. She later drafted the Hawke government's women's policy. She is author of six novels, the latest being *As the Lonely Fly*.

Jess Hill is an investigative journalist and the author of *See What You Made Me Do*. She has been a producer for ABC Radio and a journalist for Background Briefing, and Middle East correspondent for *The Global Mail*. *See What You Made Me Do* won the 2020 Stella Prize and the ABA Booksellers' Choice Adult Non-Fiction Book of the Year.

Malcolm Knox is a journalist, author and columnist for *The Sydney Morning Herald*.

Sarah Krasnostein is the multi-award-winning author of *The Trauma Cleaner* and *The Believer*. Her writing has appeared in magazines and journals in Australia, the United Kingdom and America. She holds a doctorate in criminal law.

Kieran Pender is a writer, lawyer and academic. For three years he led the International Bar Association's efforts to address sexual harassment in the legal profession. He is also a member of the advisory council of the Global Institute for Women's Leadership.

Gina Rushton is a journalist and editor, and author of *The Most Important Job in the World*.

Hannah Ryan is a journalist who has written for AAP, *Guardian Australia* and *Buzz-Feed News*, where she covered Australia's #MeToo movement. She is also a lawyer.

Amber Schultz is an associate editor and journalist at *Crikey*.

Nareen Young is professor at Jumbunna Institute of Education and Research at University of Technology, Sydney.

WANT THE LATEST FROM QUARTERLY ESSAY?

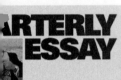
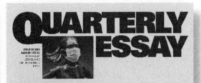
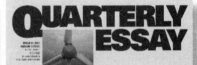

**Subscribe to the Friends of Quarterly Essay
email newsletter to share in news, updates,
events and special offers as we celebrate
our 20th anniversary.**

quarterlyessay.com.au/signup

QUARTERLY ESSAY
BACK ISSUES

BACK ISSUES: (Prices include GST, postage and handling within Australia.) *Grey indicates out of stock.*

- ☐ **QE 1** ($17.99) Robert Manne *In Denial*
- ☐ **QE 2** ($17.99) John Birmingham *Appeasing Jakarta*
- ☐ **QE 3** ($17.99) Guy Rundle *The Opportunist*
- ☐ **QE 4** ($17.99) Don Watson *Rabbit Syndrome*
- ☐ **QE 5** ($17.99) Mungo MacCallum *Girt By Sea*
- ☐ **QE 6** ($17.99) John Button *Beyond Belief*
- ☐ **QE 7** ($17.99) John Martinkus *Paradise Betrayed*
- ☐ **QE 8** ($17.99) Amanda Lohrey *Groundswell*
- ☐ **QE 9** ($17.99) Tim Flannery *Beautiful Lies*
- ☐ **QE 10** ($17.99) Gideon Haigh *Bad Company*
- ☐ **QE 11** ($17.99) Germaine Greer *Whitefella Jump Up*
- ☐ **QE 12** ($17.99) David Malouf *Made in England*
- ☐ **QE 13** ($17.99) Robert Manne with David Corlett *Sending Them Home*
- ☐ **QE 14** ($17.99) Paul McGeough *Mission Impossible*
- ☐ **QE 15** ($17.99) Margaret Simons *Latham's World*
- ☐ **QE 16** ($17.99) Raimond Gaita *Breach of Trust*
- ☐ **QE 17** ($17.99) John Hirst *'Kangaroo Court'*
- ☐ **QE 18** ($17.99) Gail Bell *The Worried Well*
- ☐ **QE 19** ($17.99) Judith Brett *Relaxed & Comfortable*
- ☐ **QE 20** ($17.99) John Birmingham *A Time for War*
- ☐ **QE 21** ($17.99) Clive Hamilton *What's Left?*
- ☐ **QE 22** ($17.99) Amanda Lohrey *Voting for Jesus*
- ☐ **QE 23** ($17.99) Inga Clendinnen *The History Question*
- ☐ **QE 24** ($17.99) Robyn Davidson *No Fixed Address*
- ☐ **QE 25** ($17.99) Peter Hartcher *Bipolar Nation*
- ☐ **QE 26** ($17.99) David Marr *His Master's Voice*
- ☐ **QE 27** ($17.99) Ian Lowe *Reaction Time*
- ☐ **QE 28** ($17.99) Judith Brett *Exit Right*
- ☐ **QE 29** ($17.99) Anne Manne *Love & Money*
- ☐ **QE 30** ($17.99) Paul Toohey *Last Drinks*
- ☐ **QE 31** ($17.99) Tim Flannery *Now or Never*
- ☐ **QE 32** ($17.99) Kate Jennings *American Revolution*
- ☐ **QE 33** ($17.99) Guy Pearse *Quarry Vision*
- ☐ **QE 34** ($17.99) Annabel Crabb *Stop at Nothing*
- ☐ **QE 35** ($17.99) Noel Pearson *Radical Hope*
- ☐ **QE 36** ($17.99) Mungo MacCallum *Australian Story*
- ☐ **QE 37** ($17.99) Waleed Aly *What's Right?*
- ☐ **QE 38** ($17.99) David Marr *Power Trip*
- ☐ **QE 39** ($17.99) Hugh White *Power Shift*
- ☐ **QE 40** ($17.99) George Megalogenis *Trivial Pursuit*
- ☐ **QE 41** ($17.99) David Malouf *The Happy Life*
- ☐ **QE 42** ($17.99) Judith Brett *Fair Share*
- ☐ **QE 43** ($17.99) Robert Manne *Bad News*
- ☐ **QE 44** ($17.99) Andrew Charlton *Man-Made World*
- ☐ **QE 45** ($17.99) Anna Krien *Us and Them*
- ☐ **QE 46** ($17.99) Laura Tingle *Great Expectations*
- ☐ **QE 47** ($17.99) David Marr *Political Animal*
- ☐ **QE 48** ($17.99) Tim Flannery *After the Future*
- ☐ **QE 49** ($17.99) Mark Latham *Not Dead Yet*
- ☐ **QE 50** ($17.99) Anna Goldsworthy *Unfinished Business*
- ☐ **QE 51** ($17.99) David Marr *The Prince*
- ☐ **QE 52** ($17.99) Linda Jaivin *Found in Translation*
- ☐ **QE 53** ($17.99) Paul Toohey *That Sinking Feeling*
- ☐ **QE 54** ($17.99) Andrew Charlton *Dragon's Tail*
- ☐ **QE 55** ($17.99) Noel Pearson *A Rightful Place*
- ☐ **QE 56** ($17.99) Guy Rundle *Clivosaurus*
- ☐ **QE 57** ($17.99) Karen Hitchcock *Dear Life*
- ☐ **QE 58** ($17.99) David Kilcullen *Blood Year*
- ☐ **QE 59** ($17.99) David Marr *Faction Man*
- ☐ **QE 60** ($17.99) Laura Tingle *Political Amnesia*
- ☐ **QE 61** ($17.99) George Megalogenis *Balancing Act*
- ☐ **QE 62** ($17.99) James Brown *Firing Line*
- ☐ **QE 63** ($17.99) Don Watson *Enemy Within*
- ☐ **QE 64** ($17.99) Stan Grant *The Australian Dream*
- ☐ **QE 65** ($17.99) David Marr *The White Queen*
- ☐ **QE 66** ($17.99) Anna Krien *The Long Goodbye*
- ☐ **QE 67** ($17.99) Benjamin Law *Moral Panic 101*
- ☐ **QE 68** ($17.99) Hugh White *Without America*
- ☐ **QE 69** ($17.99) Mark McKenna *Moment of Truth*
- ☐ **QE 70** ($17.99) Richard Denniss *Dead Right*
- ☐ **QE 71** ($17.99) Laura Tingle *Follow the Leader*
- ☐ **QE 72** ($17.99) Sebastian Smee *Net Loss*
- ☐ **QE 73** ($17.99) Rebecca Huntley *Australia Fair*
- ☐ **QE 74** ($17.99) Erik Jensen *The Prosperity Gospel*
- ☐ **QE 75** ($17.99) Annabel Crabb *Men at Work*
- ☐ **QE 76** ($17.99) Peter Hartcher *Red Flag*
- ☐ **QE 77** ($17.99) Margaret Simons *Cry Me a River*
- ☐ **QE 78** ($17.99) Judith Brett *The Coal Curse*
- ☐ **QE 79** ($17.99) Katharine Murphy *The End of Certainty*
- ☐ **QE 80** ($17.99) Laura Tingle *The High Road*
- ☐ **QE 81** ($17.99) Alan Finkel *Getting to Zero*
- ☐ **QE 82** ($24.99) George Megalogenis *Exit Strategy*
- ☐ **QE 83** ($24.99) Lech Blaine *Top Blokes*
- ☐ **QE 84** ($24.99) Jess Hill *The Reckoning*

Please include this form with delivery and payment details overleaf.
Back issues also available as eBooks at **quarterlyessay.com**

SUBSCRIBE TO RECEIVE
10% OFF THE COVER PRICE

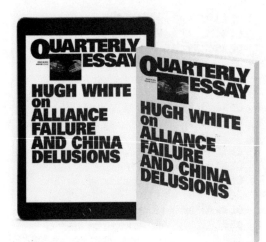

☐ **ONE-YEAR PRINT AND DIGITAL SUBSCRIPTION: $89.99**

- Print edition × 4
- Home delivery
- Full digital access to all past issues, including downloadable eBook files
- Access iPad & iPhone app
- Access Android app

DELIVERY AND PAYMENT DETAILS

DELIVERY DETAILS:

NAME:

ADDRESS:

EMAIL: PHONE:

PAYMENT DETAILS: Enclose a cheque/money order made out to Schwartz Books Pty Ltd.
Or debit my credit card (MasterCard, Visa and Amex accepted).
Freepost: Quarterly Essay, Reply Paid 90094, Collingwood VIC 3066
All prices include GST, postage and handling.

CARD NO. ☐☐☐☐ ☐☐☐☐ ☐☐☐☐ ☐☐☐☐

EXPIRY DATE: /   CCV: AMOUNT: $

PURCHASER'S NAME: SIGNATURE:

Subscribe online at **quarterlyessay.com/subscribe** • Freecall: 1800 077 514 • Phone: 03 9486 0288
Email: subscribe@quarterlyessay.com (please do not send electronic scans of this form)